Make Yourself a priority!

THIS JOURNAL belongs to _____

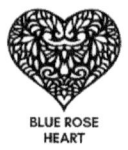

BLUE ROSE
HEART

© 2021 Blue Rose Heart Publishing. All rights reserved. No part of this publication may be reproduced, distributed or transmitted, in any form or by any means, including photocopying, recording or other electronic or mechanic methods.

WHAT IS WELLNESS?

Wellness is the act of practicing healthy habits on a daily basis to attain better physical and mental health outcomes.

By making simple and healthy choices on a daily basis, you will be well on your way towards reducing stress and achieving wellness.

Start with small changes within each area and take it one day at a time.

This journal contains a motivational quote every week and daily trackers to help you to improve:

- **Sleep:** Consider calm activities before going to bed, and wake up at the same time every day
- **Diet and nutrition:** By adding wholesome ingredients to your plate, you'll be taking steps towards becoming a healthier you
- **Physical Exercises and Mindfulness Activities:** Even 20 or 30 minutes of daily exercise can have a positive impact on your overall sense of well-being and help improve your mood. Practicing mindfulness is good for the body and mind, helps with focus and also changes the brain
- **Mood tracker:** Notice your highs and lows during the week
- **Personal activities – Hobbies:** Take some time to do something you enjoy

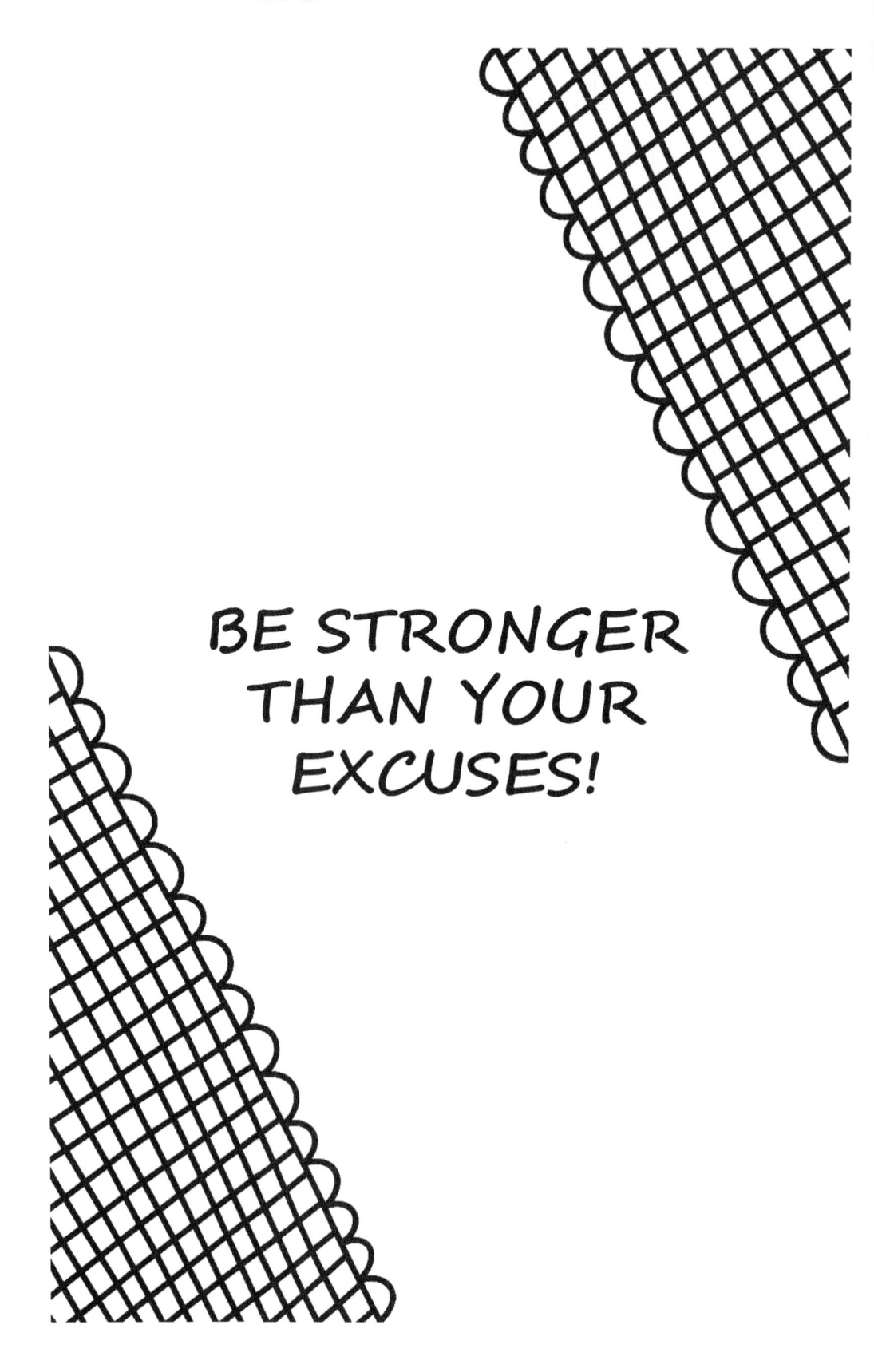

Weekly Check

WEEK	SLEEP HRS	WEIGHT	CLOTHING SIZE	OVERALL MOOD	RATE YOUR OVERALL WELLNESS (1-10)
1					
2					
3					
4					
5					
6					
7					
8					
9					
10					
11					
12					
13					
14					

Notes: _____

Date:_____

Wake Up	Bed Time	Sleep (HRS)

Diet and Nutrition – Your Food Intake

Breakfast	Lunch
Cal/Pts:	Cal/Pts:
Dinner	**Snack**
Cal/Pts:	Cal/Pts:

Water Intake

How I'm Feeling Today

Physical Exercises and Mindfulness Activities

10 20 30 40 50 60 70 80 90   ☐ Aerobic ☐ _____

Time	Intensity/Weights	Activity

Personal activities – Hobbies

_____

_____

Notes: _____

Date:_____

Wake Up	Bed Time	Sleep (HRS)

Diet and Nutrition – Your Food Intake

Breakfast	Lunch
Cal/Pts:	Cal/Pts:
Dinner	**Snack**
Cal/Pts:	Cal/Pts:

Water Intake

How I'm Feeling Today

Physical Exercises and Mindfulness Activities

10 20 30 40 50 60 70 80 90   ☐ Aerobic   ☐ _____

Time	Intensity/Weights	Activity

Personal activities – Hobbies

_____

_____

Notes: _____

Date:_____

Wake Up	Bed Time	Sleep (HRS)

Diet and Nutrition – Your Food Intake

Breakfast	Lunch
Cal/Pts:	Cal/Pts:
Dinner	**Snack**
Cal/Pts:	Cal/Pts:

Water Intake   How I'm Feeling Today

Physical Exercises and Mindfulness Activities

10 20 30 40 50 60 70 80 90   ☐ Aerobic   ☐ _____

Time	Intensity/Weights	Activity

Personal activities – Hobbies

_____

_____

Notes: _____

Date:_____

Wake Up	Bed Time	Sleep (HRS)

Diet and Nutrition – Your Food Intake

Breakfast	Lunch
Cal/Pts:	Cal/Pts:
Dinner	**Snack**
Cal/Pts:	Cal/Pts:

Water Intake

How I'm Feeling Today

Physical Exercises and Mindfulness Activities

10 20 30 40 50 60 70 80 90 ☐ Aerobic ☐ _____

Time	Intensity/Weights	Activity

Personal activities – Hobbies

_____
_____

Notes: _____
_____

Date:_____

Wake Up	Bed Time	Sleep (HRS)

Diet and Nutrition – Your Food Intake

Breakfast	Lunch
Cal/Pts:	Cal/Pts:
Dinner	**Snack**
Cal/Pts:	Cal/Pts:

Water Intake

How I'm Feeling Today

Physical Exercises and Mindfulness Activities

10 20 30 40 50 60 70 80 90   ☐ Aerobic   ☐ _____

Time	Intensity/Weights	Activity

Personal activities – Hobbies

_____
_____

Notes: _____
_____

Date:_____

Wake Up	Bed Time	Sleep (HRS)

Diet and Nutrition – Your Food Intake

Breakfast	Lunch
Cal/Pts:	Cal/Pts:
Dinner	**Snack**
Cal/Pts:	Cal/Pts:

Water Intake

How I'm Feeling Today

Physical Exercises and Mindfulness Activities

10 20 30 40 50 60 70 80 90   ☐ Aerobic ☐ _____

Time	Intensity/Weights	Activity

Personal activities – Hobbies

_____
_____

Notes: _____

Date:_____

Wake Up	Bed Time	Sleep (HRS)

Diet and Nutrition – Your Food Intake

Breakfast	Lunch
Cal/Pts:	Cal/Pts:
Dinner	**Snack**
Cal/Pts:	Cal/Pts:

Water Intake

How I'm Feeling Today

Physical Exercises and Mindfulness Activities

10 20 30 40 50 60 70 80 90   ☐ Aerobic ☐ _____

Time	Intensity/Weights	Activity

Personal activities – Hobbies

_____

_____

Notes: _____

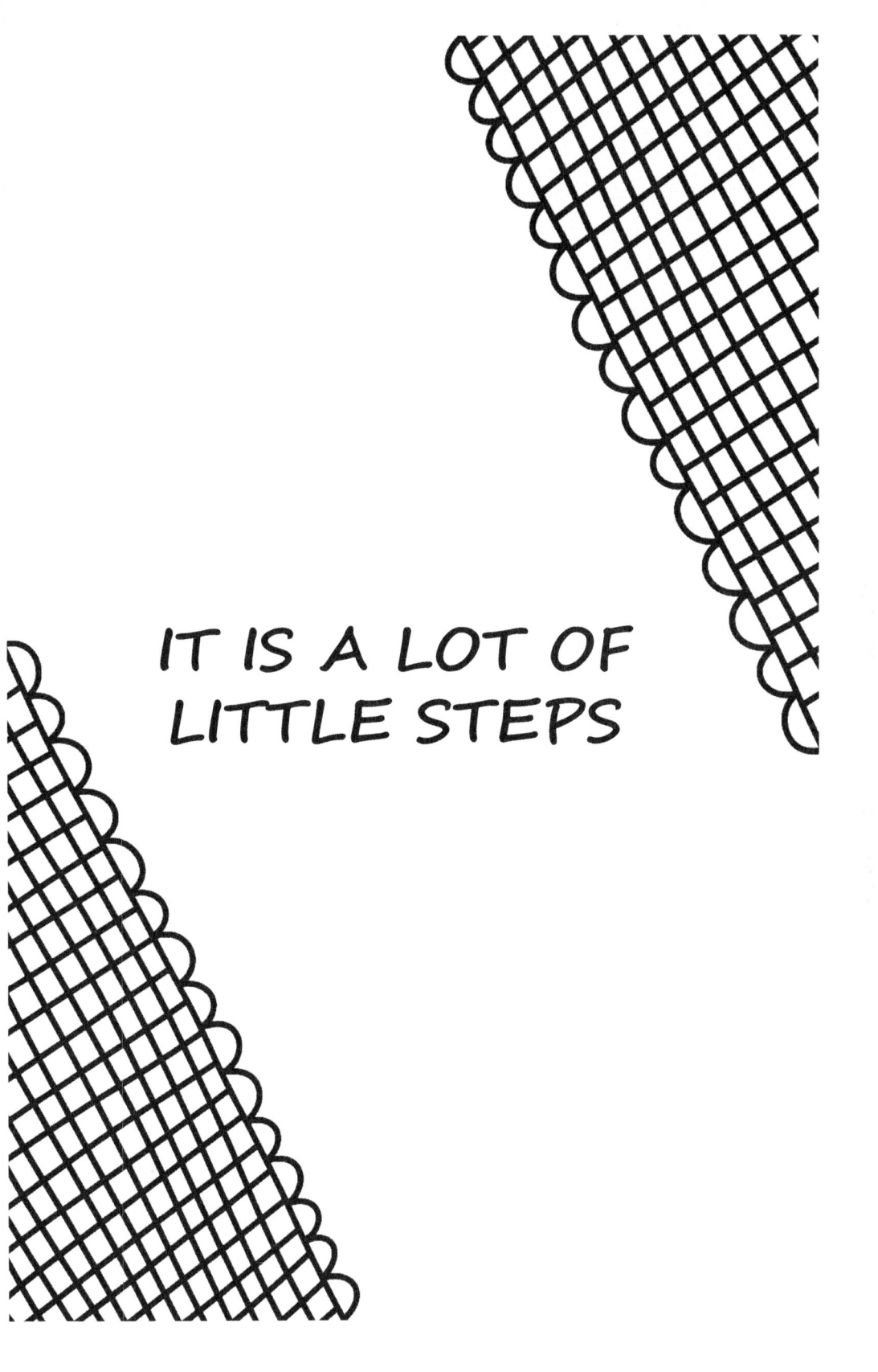

Date:_____

Wake Up	Bed Time	Sleep (HRS)

Diet and Nutrition – Your Food Intake

Breakfast	Lunch
Cal/Pts:	Cal/Pts:
Dinner	**Snack**
Cal/Pts:	Cal/Pts:

Water Intake

How I'm Feeling Today

Physical Exercises and Mindfulness Activities

10 20 30 40 50 60 70 80 90   ☐ Aerobic ☐ _____

Time	Intensity/Weights	Activity

Personal activities – Hobbies

_____

_____

Notes: _____

Date:_____

Wake Up	Bed Time	Sleep (HRS)

Diet and Nutrition – Your Food Intake

Breakfast	Lunch
Cal/Pts:	Cal/Pts:
Dinner	**Snack**
Cal/Pts:	Cal/Pts:

Water Intake

How I'm Feeling Today

Physical Exercises and Mindfulness Activities

10 20 30 40 50 60 70 80 90   ☐ Aerobic   ☐ _____

Time	Intensity/Weights	Activity

Personal activities – Hobbies

_____
_____

Notes: _____
_____

Date:_____

Wake Up	Bed Time	Sleep (HRS)

Diet and Nutrition – Your Food Intake

Breakfast	Lunch
Cal/Pts:	Cal/Pts:
Dinner	**Snack**
Cal/Pts:	Cal/Pts:

Water Intake   How I'm Feeling Today

Physical Exercises and Mindfulness Activities

10 20 30 40 50 60 70 80 90   ☐ Aerobic   ☐ _____

Time	Intensity/Weights	Activity

Personal activities – Hobbies

_____
_____

Notes: _____
_____

Date:_____

Wake Up	Bed Time	Sleep (HRS)

Diet and Nutrition – Your Food Intake

Breakfast	Lunch
Cal/Pts:	Cal/Pts:
Dinner	**Snack**
Cal/Pts:	Cal/Pts:

Water Intake

How I'm Feeling Today

Physical Exercises and Mindfulness Activities

10 20 30 40 50 60 70 80 90   ☐ Aerobic   ☐ _____

Time	Intensity/Weights	Activity

Personal activities – Hobbies

_____
_____

Notes: _____
_____

Date:_____

Wake Up	Bed Time	Sleep (HRS)

Diet and Nutrition – Your Food Intake

Breakfast	Lunch
Cal/Pts:	Cal/Pts:
Dinner	**Snack**
Cal/Pts:	Cal/Pts:

Water Intake

How I'm Feeling Today

Physical Exercises and Mindfulness Activities

10 20 30 40 50 60 70 80 90   ☐ Aerobic   ☐ _____

Time	Intensity/Weights	Activity

Personal activities – Hobbies

_____

_____

Notes: _____

Date:_____

Wake Up	Bed Time	Sleep (HRS)

Diet and Nutrition – Your Food Intake

Breakfast	Lunch
Cal/Pts:	Cal/Pts:
Dinner	**Snack**
Cal/Pts:	Cal/Pts:

Water Intake

How I'm Feeling Today

Physical Exercises and Mindfulness Activities

10 20 30 40 50 60 70 80 90   ☐ Aerobic   ☐ _____

Time	Intensity/Weights	Activity

Personal activities – Hobbies

_____

_____

Notes: _____

Date:_____

Wake Up	Bed Time	Sleep (HRS)

Diet and Nutrition – Your Food Intake

Breakfast	Lunch
Cal/Pts:	Cal/Pts:
Dinner	**Snack**
Cal/Pts:	Cal/Pts:

Water Intake

How I'm Feeling Today

Physical Exercises and Mindfulness Activities

10 20 30 40 50 60 70 80 90   ☐ Aerobic   ☐ _____

Time	Intensity/Weights	Activity

Personal activities – Hobbies

_____

_____

Notes: _____

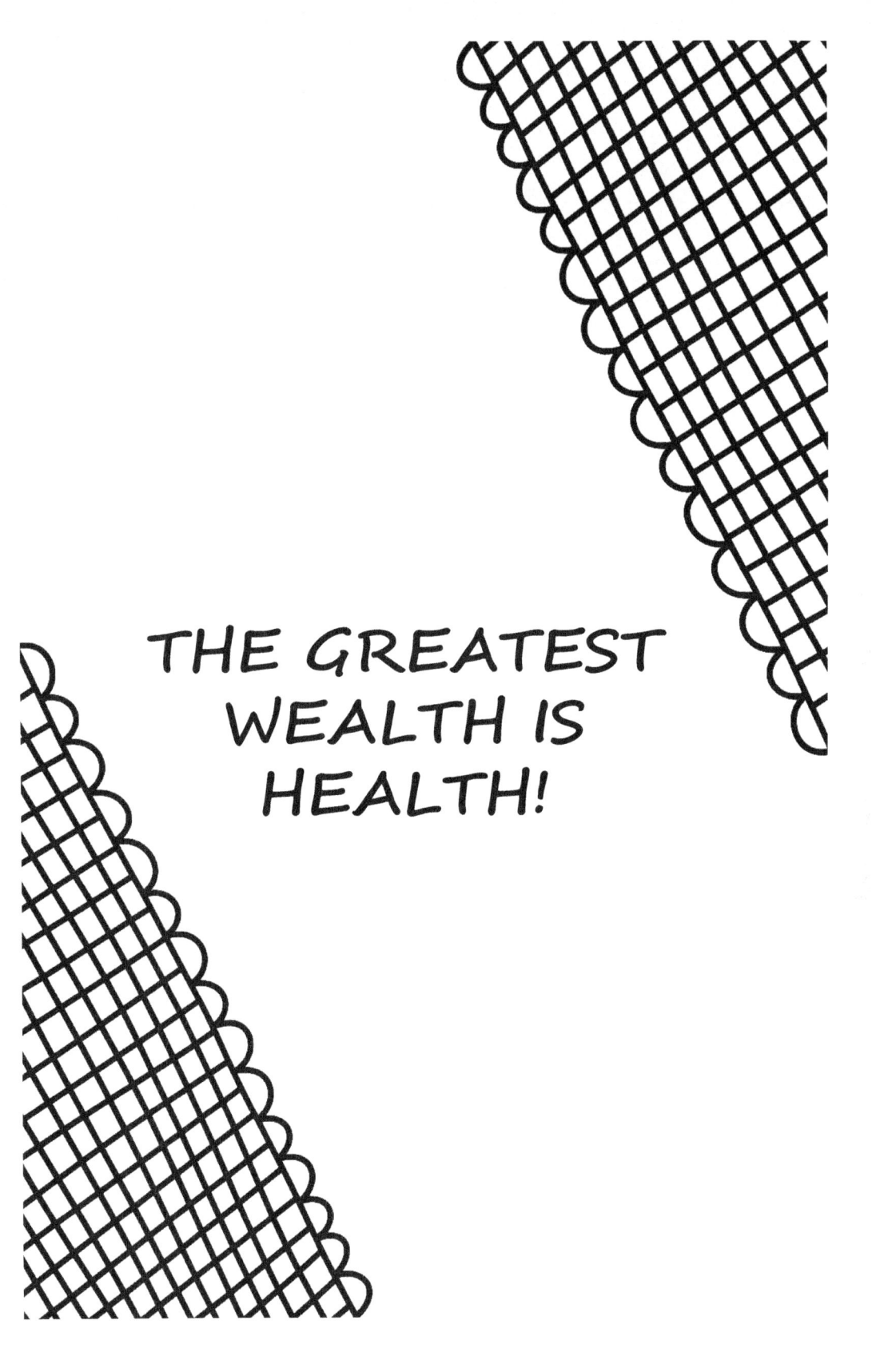

Date:_____

Wake Up	Bed Time	Sleep (HRS)

Diet and Nutrition – Your Food Intake

Breakfast	Lunch
Cal/Pts:	Cal/Pts:
Dinner	**Snack**
Cal/Pts:	Cal/Pts:

Water Intake

How I'm Feeling Today

Physical Exercises and Mindfulness Activities

10 20 30 40 50 60 70 80 90   ☐ Aerobic   ☐ _____

Time	Intensity/Weights	Activity

Personal activities – Hobbies

_____
_____

Notes: _____

Date:_____

Wake Up	Bed Time	Sleep (HRS)

Diet and Nutrition – Your Food Intake

Breakfast	Lunch
Cal/Pts:	Cal/Pts:
Dinner	**Snack**
Cal/Pts:	Cal/Pts:

Water Intake   How I'm Feeling Today

Physical Exercises and Mindfulness Activities

10 20 30 40 50 60 70 80 90 ☐ Aerobic ☐ _____

Time	Intensity/Weights	Activity

Personal activities – Hobbies

_____
_____

Notes: _____

Date:_____

Wake Up	Bed Time	Sleep (HRS)

Diet and Nutrition – Your Food Intake

Breakfast	Lunch
Cal/Pts:	Cal/Pts:
Dinner	**Snack**
Cal/Pts:	Cal/Pts:

Water Intake   How I'm Feeling Today

Physical Exercises and Mindfulness Activities

10 20 30 40 50 60 70 80 90   ☐ Aerobic   ☐ _____

Time	Intensity/Weights	Activity

Personal activities – Hobbies

_____

_____

Notes: _____

Date:_____

Wake Up	Bed Time	Sleep (HRS)

Diet and Nutrition – Your Food Intake

Breakfast	Lunch
Cal/Pts:	Cal/Pts:
Dinner	**Snack**
Cal/Pts:	Cal/Pts:

Water Intake

How I'm Feeling Today

Physical Exercises and Mindfulness Activities

10 20 30 40 50 60 70 80 90   ☐ Aerobic   ☐ _____

Time	Intensity/Weights	Activity

Personal activities – Hobbies

_____

_____

Notes: _____

Date:_____

Wake Up	Bed Time	Sleep (HRS)

Diet and Nutrition – Your Food Intake

Breakfast	Lunch
Cal/Pts:	Cal/Pts:
Dinner	**Snack**
Cal/Pts:	Cal/Pts:

Water Intake

How I'm Feeling Today

Physical Exercises and Mindfulness Activities

10 20 30 40 50 60 70 80 90   ☐ Aerobic   ☐ _____

Time	Intensity/Weights	Activity

Personal activities – Hobbies

_____

_____

Notes: _____

Date:_____

Wake Up	Bed Time	Sleep (HRS)

Diet and Nutrition – Your Food Intake

Breakfast	Lunch
Cal/Pts:	Cal/Pts:
Dinner	**Snack**
Cal/Pts:	Cal/Pts:

Water Intake

How I'm Feeling Today

Physical Exercises and Mindfulness Activities

10 20 30 40 50 60 70 80 90 ☐ Aerobic ☐ _____

Time	Intensity/Weights	Activity

Personal activities – Hobbies

_____
_____

Notes: _____
_____

Date:_____

Wake Up	Bed Time	Sleep (HRS)

Diet and Nutrition – Your Food Intake

Breakfast	Lunch
Cal/Pts:	Cal/Pts:
Dinner	**Snack**
Cal/Pts:	Cal/Pts:

Water Intake   How I'm Feeling Today

Physical Exercises and Mindfulness Activities

10 20 30 40 50 60 70 80 90 ☐ Aerobic ☐ _____

Time	Intensity/Weights	Activity

Personal activities – Hobbies

_____
_____

Notes: _____

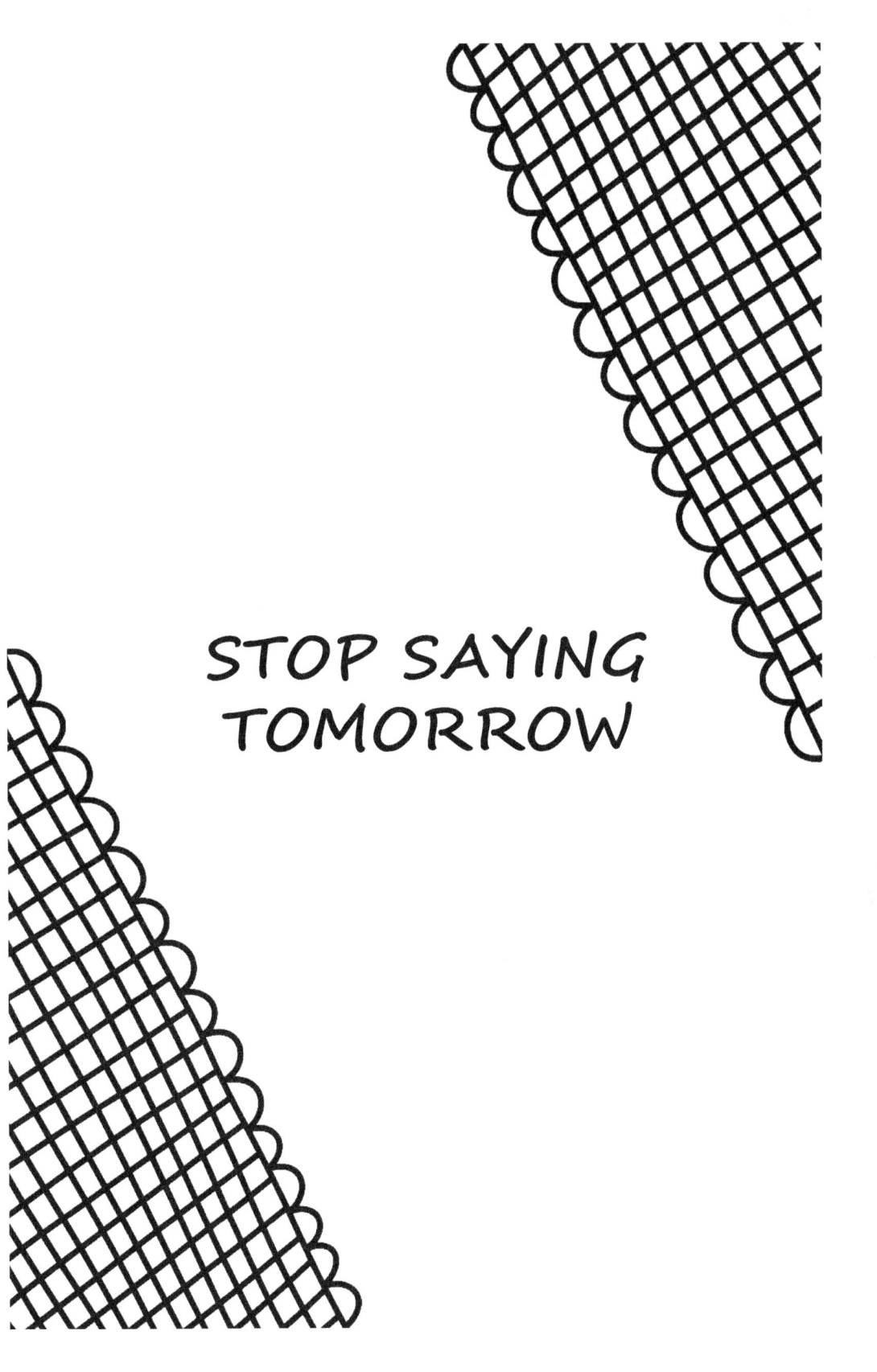

Date:_____

Wake Up	Bed Time	Sleep (HRS)

Diet and Nutrition – Your Food Intake

Breakfast	Lunch
Cal/Pts:	Cal/Pts:
Dinner	**Snack**
Cal/Pts:	Cal/Pts:

Water Intake

How I'm Feeling Today

Physical Exercises and Mindfulness Activities

10 20 30 40 50 60 70 80 90   ☐ Aerobic   ☐ _____

Time	Intensity/Weights	Activity

Personal activities – Hobbies

_____

_____

Notes: _____

Date:_____

Wake Up	Bed Time	Sleep (HRS)

Diet and Nutrition – Your Food Intake

Breakfast	Lunch
Cal/Pts:	Cal/Pts:
Dinner	**Snack**
Cal/Pts:	Cal/Pts:

Water Intake

How I'm Feeling Today

Physical Exercises and Mindfulness Activities

10 20 30 40 50 60 70 80 90   ☐ Aerobic   ☐ _____

Time	Intensity/Weights	Activity

Personal activities – Hobbies

_____

_____

Notes: _____

Date:_____

Wake Up	Bed Time	Sleep (HRS)

Diet and Nutrition – Your Food Intake

Breakfast	Lunch
Cal/Pts:	Cal/Pts:
Dinner	**Snack**
Cal/Pts:	Cal/Pts:

Water Intake

How I'm Feeling Today

Physical Exercises and Mindfulness Activities

10 20 30 40 50 60 70 80 90   ☐ Aerobic   ☐ _____

Time	Intensity/Weights	Activity

Personal activities – Hobbies

_____

_____

Notes: _____

Date:_____

Wake Up	Bed Time	Sleep (HRS)

Diet and Nutrition – Your Food Intake

Breakfast	Lunch
Cal/Pts:	Cal/Pts:
Dinner	**Snack**
Cal/Pts:	Cal/Pts:

Water Intake   How I'm Feeling Today

Physical Exercises and Mindfulness Activities

10 20 30 40 50 60 70 80 90 ☐ Aerobic ☐ _____

Time	Intensity/Weights	Activity

Personal activities – Hobbies

_____

_____

Notes: _____

_____

Date:_____

Wake Up	Bed Time	Sleep (HRS)

Diet and Nutrition – Your Food Intake

Breakfast	Lunch
Cal/Pts:	Cal/Pts:
Dinner	**Snack**
Cal/Pts:	Cal/Pts:

Water Intake   How I'm Feeling Today

Physical Exercises and Mindfulness Activities

10 20 30 40 50 60 70 80 90 ☐ Aerobic ☐ _____

Time	Intensity/Weights	Activity

Personal activities – Hobbies

_____
_____

Notes: _____

Date:_____

Wake Up	Bed Time	Sleep (HRS)

Diet and Nutrition – Your Food Intake

Breakfast	Lunch
Cal/Pts:	Cal/Pts:
Dinner	**Snack**
Cal/Pts:	Cal/Pts:

Water Intake

How I'm Feeling Today

Physical Exercises and Mindfulness Activities

10 20 30 40 50 60 70 80 90   ☐ Aerobic   ☐ _____

Time	Intensity/Weights	Activity

Personal activities – Hobbies

_____
_____

Notes: _____
_____

Date:_____

Wake Up	Bed Time	Sleep (HRS)

Diet and Nutrition – Your Food Intake

Breakfast	Lunch
Cal/Pts:	Cal/Pts:
Dinner	**Snack**
Cal/Pts:	Cal/Pts:

Water Intake

How I'm Feeling Today

Physical Exercises and Mindfulness Activities

10 20 30 40 50 60 70 80 90   ☐ Aerobic   ☐ _____

Time	Intensity/Weights	Activity

Personal activities – Hobbies

_____

_____

Notes: _____

BELIEVE IN YOURSELF!

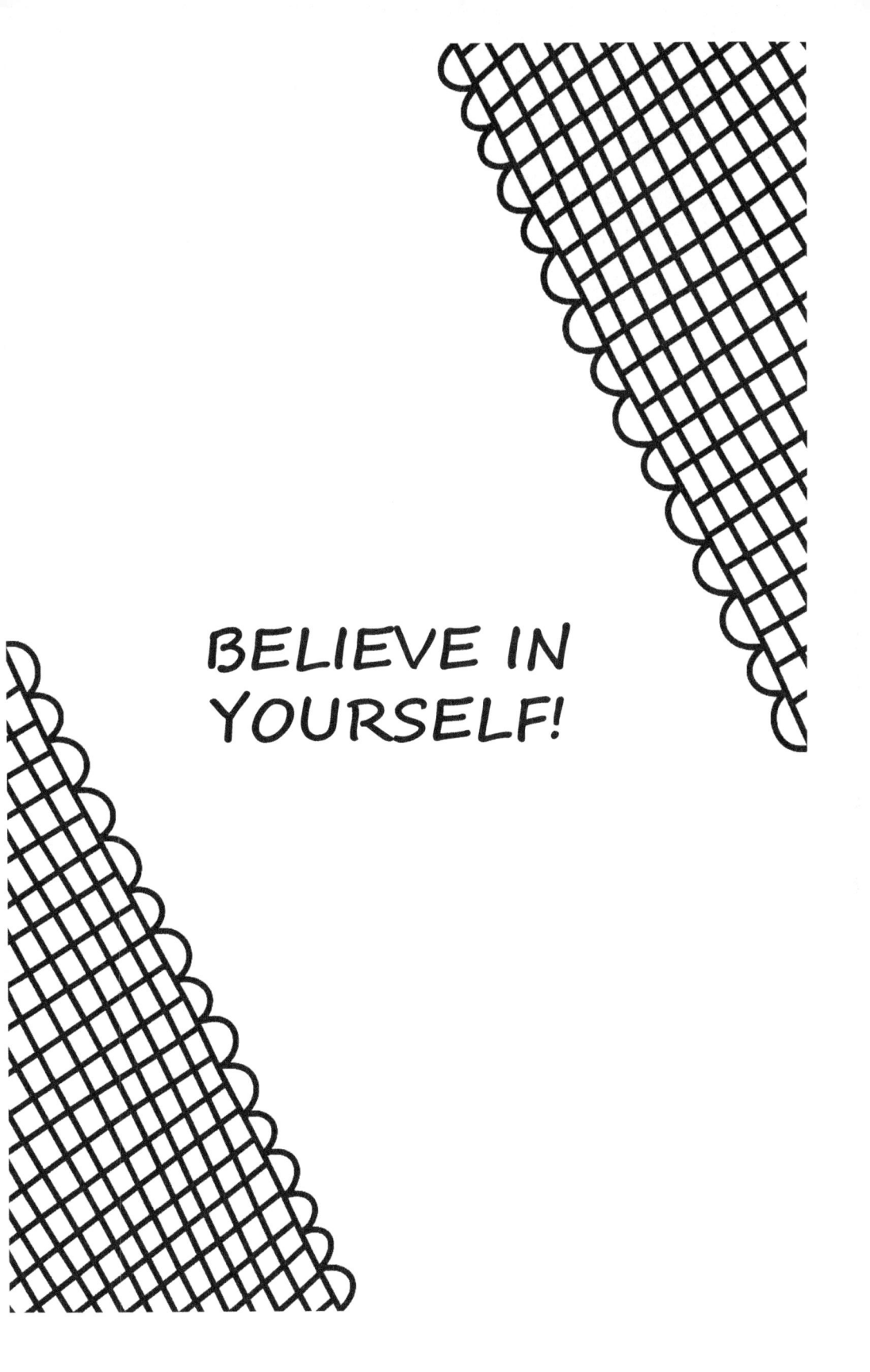

Date:_____

Wake Up	Bed Time	Sleep (HRS)

Diet and Nutrition – Your Food Intake

Breakfast	Lunch
Cal/Pts:	Cal/Pts:
Dinner	**Snack**
Cal/Pts:	Cal/Pts:

Water Intake   How I'm Feeling Today

Physical Exercises and Mindfulness Activities

10 20 30 40 50 60 70 80 90   ☐ Aerobic   ☐ _____

Time	Intensity/Weights	Activity

Personal activities – Hobbies

_____

_____

Notes: _____
_____

Date:_____

Wake Up	Bed Time	Sleep (HRS)

Diet and Nutrition – Your Food Intake

Breakfast	Lunch
Cal/Pts:	Cal/Pts:
Dinner	**Snack**
Cal/Pts:	Cal/Pts:

Water Intake

How I'm Feeling Today

Physical Exercises and Mindfulness Activities

10 20 30 40 50 60 70 80 90   ☐ Aerobic   ☐ _____

Time	Intensity/Weights	Activity

Personal activities – Hobbies

_____
_____

Notes: _____
_____

Date:_____

Wake Up	Bed Time	Sleep (HRS)

Diet and Nutrition – Your Food Intake

Breakfast	Lunch
Cal/Pts:	Cal/Pts:
Dinner	**Snack**
Cal/Pts:	Cal/Pts:

Water Intake   How I'm Feeling Today

Physical Exercises and Mindfulness Activities

10 20 30 40 50 60 70 80 90   ☐ Aerobic   ☐ _____

Time	Intensity/Weights	Activity

Personal activities – Hobbies

_____
_____

Notes: _____
_____

Date:_____

Wake Up	Bed Time	Sleep (HRS)

Diet and Nutrition – Your Food Intake

Breakfast	Lunch
Cal/Pts:	Cal/Pts:
Dinner	**Snack**
Cal/Pts:	Cal/Pts:

Water Intake

How I'm Feeling Today

Physical Exercises and Mindfulness Activities

10 20 30 40 50 60 70 80 90 ☐ Aerobic ☐ _____

Time	Intensity/Weights	Activity

Personal activities – Hobbies

_____
_____

Notes: _____

Date:_____

Wake Up	Bed Time	Sleep (HRS)

Diet and Nutrition – Your Food Intake

Breakfast	Lunch
Cal/Pts:	Cal/Pts:
Dinner	**Snack**
Cal/Pts:	Cal/Pts:

Water Intake

How I'm Feeling Today

Physical Exercises and Mindfulness Activities

10 20 30 40 50 60 70 80 90   ☐ Aerobic   ☐ _____

Time	Intensity/Weights	Activity

Personal activities – Hobbies

_____

_____

Notes: _____

Date:_____

Wake Up	Bed Time	Sleep (HRS)

Diet and Nutrition – Your Food Intake

Breakfast	Lunch
Cal/Pts:	Cal/Pts:
Dinner	**Snack**
Cal/Pts:	Cal/Pts:

Water Intake

How I'm Feeling Today

Physical Exercises and Mindfulness Activities

10 20 30 40 50 60 70 80 90 ☐ Aerobic ☐ _____

Time	Intensity/Weights	Activity

Personal activities – Hobbies

_____

_____

Notes: _____

Date:_____

Wake Up	Bed Time	Sleep (HRS)

Diet and Nutrition – Your Food Intake

Breakfast	Lunch
Cal/Pts:	Cal/Pts:
Dinner	**Snack**
Cal/Pts:	Cal/Pts:

Water Intake   How I'm Feeling Today

Physical Exercises and Mindfulness Activities

10 20 30 40 50 60 70 80 90   ☐ Aerobic   ☐ _____

Time	Intensity/Weights	Activity

Personal activities – Hobbies

_____
_____

Notes: _____

BUILD GOOD HABITS!

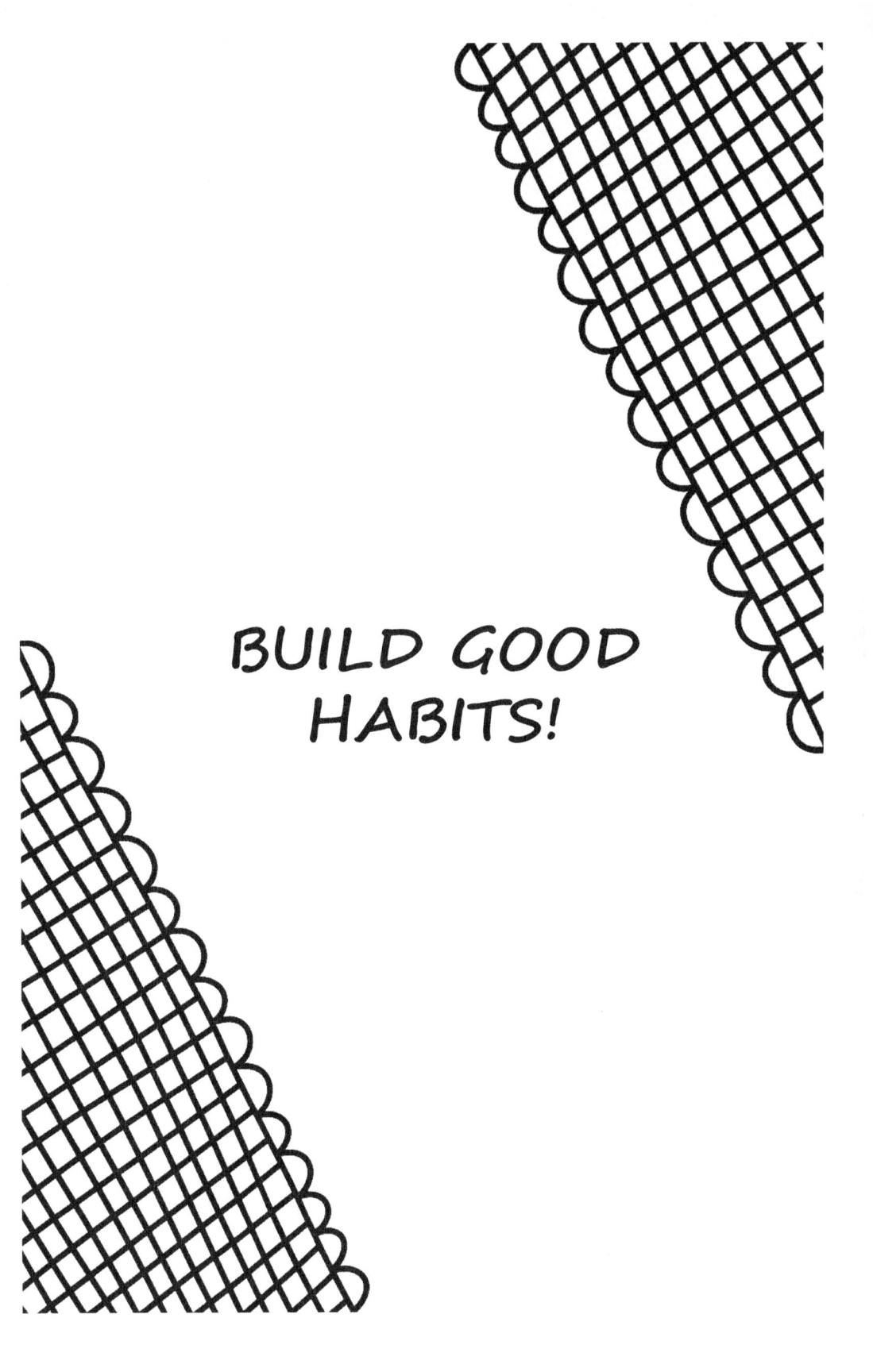

Date:_____

Wake Up	Bed Time	Sleep (HRS)

Diet and Nutrition – Your Food Intake

Breakfast	Lunch
Cal/Pts:	Cal/Pts:
Dinner	**Snack**
Cal/Pts:	Cal/Pts:

Water Intake   How I'm Feeling Today

Physical Exercises and Mindfulness Activities

10 20 30 40 50 60 70 80 90   ☐ Aerobic   ☐ _____

Time	Intensity/Weights	Activity

Personal activities – Hobbies

_____
_____

Notes: _____
_____

Date:_____

Wake Up	Bed Time	Sleep (HRS)

Diet and Nutrition – Your Food Intake

Breakfast	Lunch
Cal/Pts:	Cal/Pts:
Dinner	**Snack**
Cal/Pts:	Cal/Pts:

Water Intake 　　　　　　　How I'm Feeling Today

Physical Exercises and Mindfulness Activities

10 20 30 40 50 60 70 80 90   ☐ Aerobic   ☐ _____

Time	Intensity/Weights	Activity

Personal activities – Hobbies

_____
_____

Notes: _____
_____

Date:_____

Wake Up	Bed Time	Sleep (HRS)

Diet and Nutrition – Your Food Intake

Breakfast	Lunch
Cal/Pts:	Cal/Pts:
Dinner	**Snack**
Cal/Pts:	Cal/Pts:

Water Intake

How I'm Feeling Today

Physical Exercises and Mindfulness Activities

10 20 30 40 50 60 70 80 90   ☐ Aerobic ☐ _____

Time	Intensity/Weights	Activity

Personal activities – Hobbies

_____

_____

Notes: _____

Date:_____

Wake Up	Bed Time	Sleep (HRS)

Diet and Nutrition – Your Food Intake

Breakfast	Lunch
Cal/Pts:	Cal/Pts:
Dinner	**Snack**
Cal/Pts:	Cal/Pts:

Water Intake

How I'm Feeling Today

Physical Exercises and Mindfulness Activities

10 20 30 40 50 60 70 80 90   ☐ Aerobic   ☐ _____

Time	Intensity/Weights	Activity

Personal activities – Hobbies

_____
_____

Notes: _____

Date:_____

Wake Up	Bed Time	Sleep (HRS)

Diet and Nutrition – Your Food Intake

Breakfast	Lunch
Cal/Pts:	Cal/Pts:
Dinner	**Snack**
Cal/Pts:	Cal/Pts:

Water Intake   How I'm Feeling Today

Physical Exercises and Mindfulness Activities

10 20 30 40 50 60 70 80 90   ☐ Aerobic   ☐ _____

Time	Intensity/Weights	Activity

Personal activities – Hobbies

_____
_____

Notes: _____
       _____

Date:_____

Wake Up	Bed Time	Sleep (HRS)

Diet and Nutrition – Your Food Intake

Breakfast	Lunch
Cal/Pts:	Cal/Pts:
Dinner	**Snack**
Cal/Pts:	Cal/Pts:

Water Intake   How I'm Feeling Today

Physical Exercises and Mindfulness Activities

10 20 30 40 50 60 70 80 90   ☐ Aerobic   ☐ _____

Time	Intensity/Weights	Activity

Personal activities – Hobbies

_____

_____

Notes: _____

Date:_____

Wake Up	Bed Time	Sleep (HRS)

Diet and Nutrition – Your Food Intake

Breakfast	Lunch
  Cal/Pts:	 Cal/Pts:
Dinner	**Snack**
  Cal/Pts:	 Cal/Pts:

Water Intake

How I'm Feeling Today

Physical Exercises and Mindfulness Activities

10 20 30 40 50 60 70 80 90   ☐ Aerobic   ☐ _____

Time	Intensity/Weights	Activity

Personal activities – Hobbies

_____
_____

Notes: _____

POSITIVE THINKING! POSITIVE OUTCOME!

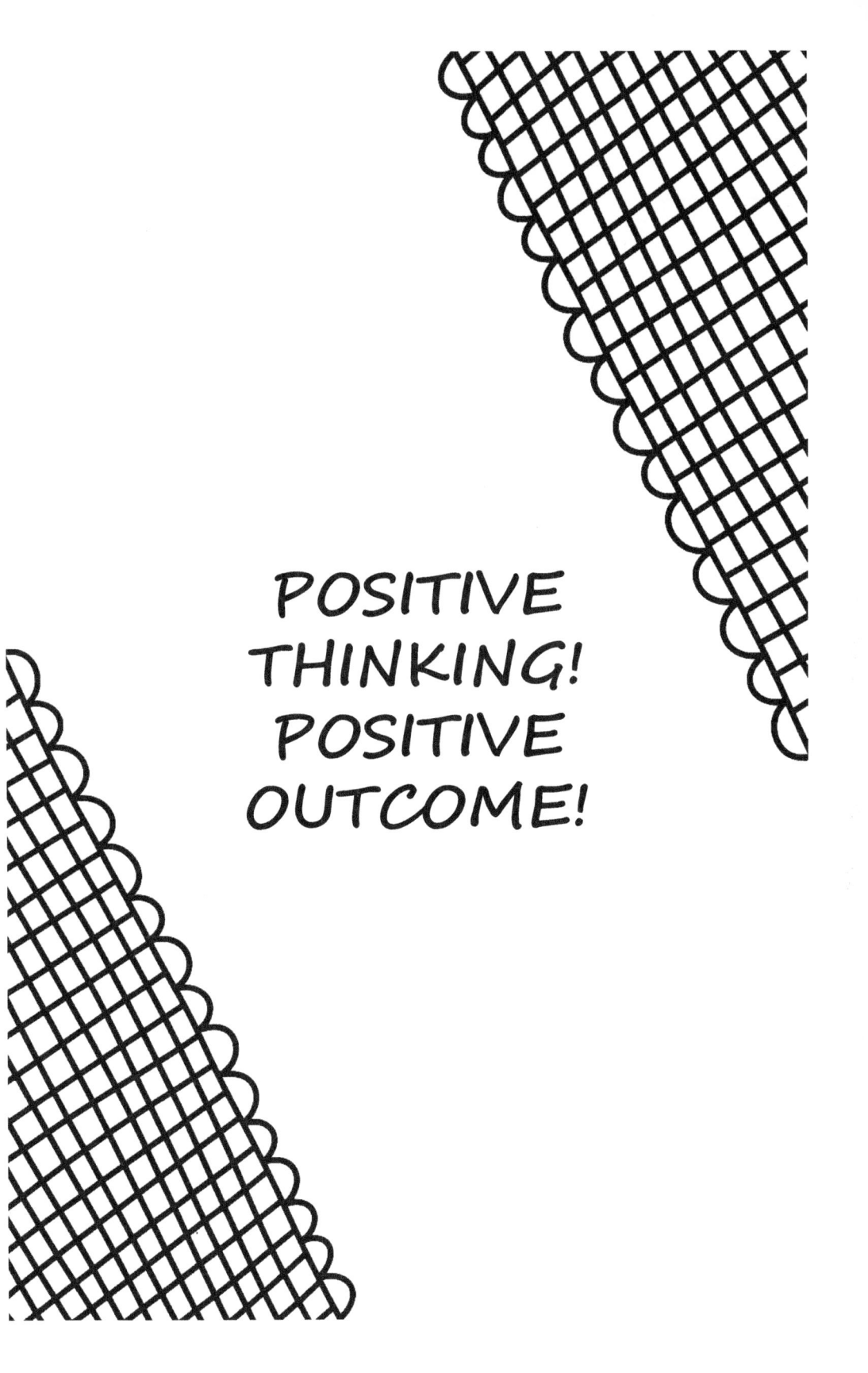

Date:_____

Wake Up	Bed Time	Sleep (HRS)

Diet and Nutrition – Your Food Intake

Breakfast	Lunch
Cal/Pts:	Cal/Pts:
Dinner	**Snack**
Cal/Pts:	Cal/Pts:

Water Intake

How I'm Feeling Today

Physical Exercises and Mindfulness Activities

10 20 30 40 50 60 70 80 90   ☐ Aerobic   ☐ _____

Time	Intensity/Weights	Activity

Personal activities – Hobbies

_____

_____

Notes: _____
_____

Date:_____

Wake Up	Bed Time	Sleep (HRS)

Diet and Nutrition – Your Food Intake

Breakfast	Lunch
Cal/Pts:	Cal/Pts:
Dinner	**Snack**
Cal/Pts:	Cal/Pts:

Water Intake

How I'm Feeling Today

Physical Exercises and Mindfulness Activities

10 20 30 40 50 60 70 80 90   ☐ Aerobic ☐ _____

Time	Intensity/Weights	Activity

Personal activities – Hobbies

_____

_____

Notes: _____

Date:_____

Wake Up	Bed Time	Sleep (HRS)

Diet and Nutrition – Your Food Intake

Breakfast	Lunch
Cal/Pts:	Cal/Pts:

Dinner	Snack
Cal/Pts:	Cal/Pts:

Water Intake

How I'm Feeling Today

Physical Exercises and Mindfulness Activities

10 20 30 40 50 60 70 80 90   ☐ Aerobic ☐ _____

Time	Intensity/Weights	Activity

Personal activities – Hobbies

_____

_____

Notes: _____

Date:_____

Wake Up	Bed Time	Sleep (HRS)

Diet and Nutrition – Your Food Intake

Breakfast	Lunch
Cal/Pts:	Cal/Pts:
Dinner	**Snack**
Cal/Pts:	Cal/Pts:

Water Intake

How I'm Feeling Today

Physical Exercises and Mindfulness Activities

10 20 30 40 50 60 70 80 90   ☐ Aerobic   ☐ _____

Time	Intensity/Weights	Activity

Personal activities – Hobbies

_____

_____

Notes: _____

Date:_____

Wake Up	Bed Time	Sleep (HRS)

Diet and Nutrition – Your Food Intake

Breakfast	Lunch
Cal/Pts:	Cal/Pts:
Dinner	**Snack**
Cal/Pts:	Cal/Pts:

Water Intake

How I'm Feeling Today

Physical Exercises and Mindfulness Activities

10 20 30 40 50 60 70 80 90   ☐ Aerobic   ☐ _____

Time	Intensity/Weights	Activity

Personal activities – Hobbies

_____
_____

Notes: _____
_____

Date:_____

Wake Up	Bed Time	Sleep (HRS)

Diet and Nutrition – Your Food Intake

Breakfast	Lunch
Cal/Pts:	Cal/Pts:
Dinner	**Snack**
Cal/Pts:	Cal/Pts:

Water Intake

How I'm Feeling Today

Physical Exercises and Mindfulness Activities

10 20 30 40 50 60 70 80 90   ☐ Aerobic   ☐ _____

Time	Intensity/Weights	Activity

Personal activities – Hobbies

_____
_____

Notes: _____
_____

Date:_____

Wake Up	Bed Time	Sleep (HRS)

Diet and Nutrition – Your Food Intake

Breakfast	Lunch
Cal/Pts:	Cal/Pts:
Dinner	**Snack**
Cal/Pts:	Cal/Pts:

Water Intake   How I'm Feeling Today

Physical Exercises and Mindfulness Activities

10 20 30 40 50 60 70 80 90 ☐ Aerobic ☐ _____

Time	Intensity/Weights	Activity

Personal activities – Hobbies

_____

_____

Notes: _____

SLOW PROGRESS IS BETTER THAN NO PROGRESS!

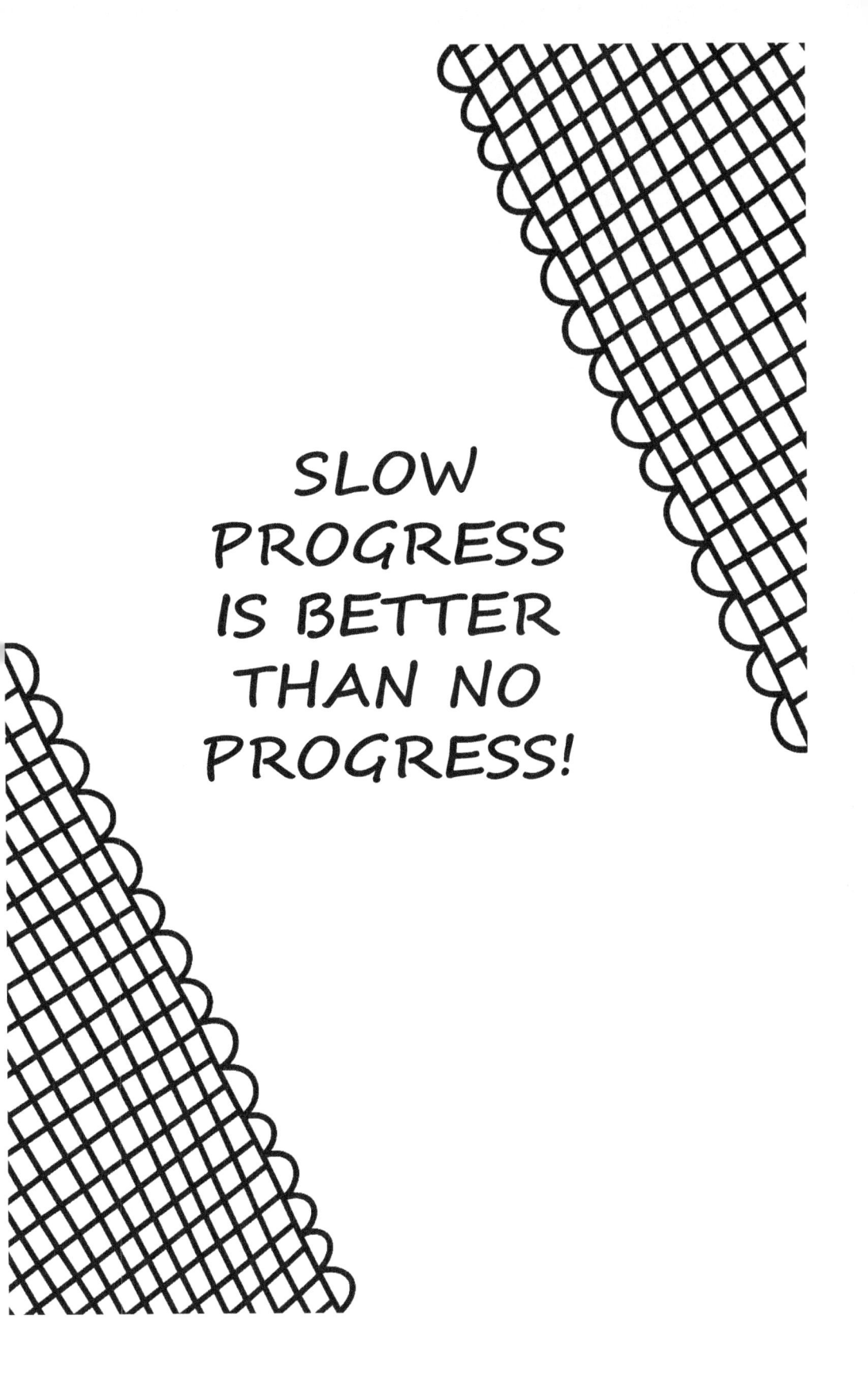

Date:_____

Wake Up	Bed Time	Sleep (HRS)

Diet and Nutrition – Your Food Intake

Breakfast	Lunch
Cal/Pts:	Cal/Pts:
Dinner	**Snack**
Cal/Pts:	Cal/Pts:

Water Intake   How I'm Feeling Today

Physical Exercises and Mindfulness Activities

10 20 30 40 50 60 70 80 90   ☐ Aerobic   ☐ _____

Time	Intensity/Weights	Activity

Personal activities – Hobbies

_____

_____

Notes: _____

_____

Date:_____

Wake Up	Bed Time	Sleep (HRS)

Diet and Nutrition – Your Food Intake

Breakfast	Lunch
Cal/Pts:	Cal/Pts:
Dinner	**Snack**
Cal/Pts:	Cal/Pts:

Water Intake

How I'm Feeling Today

Physical Exercises and Mindfulness Activities

10 20 30 40 50 60 70 80 90   ☐ Aerobic   ☐ _____

Time	Intensity/Weights	Activity

Personal activities – Hobbies

_____

_____

Notes: _____

Date:_____

Wake Up	Bed Time	Sleep (HRS)

Diet and Nutrition – Your Food Intake

Breakfast	Lunch
Cal/Pts:	Cal/Pts:
Dinner	**Snack**
Cal/Pts:	Cal/Pts:

Water Intake   How I'm Feeling Today

Physical Exercises and Mindfulness Activities

10 20 30 40 50 60 70 80 90   ☐ Aerobic   ☐ _____

Time	Intensity/Weights	Activity

Personal activities – Hobbies

_____
_____

Notes: _____
_____

Date:_____

Wake Up	Bed Time	Sleep (HRS)

Diet and Nutrition – Your Food Intake

Breakfast	Lunch
Cal/Pts:	Cal/Pts:
Dinner	**Snack**
Cal/Pts:	Cal/Pts:

Water Intake

How I'm Feeling Today

Physical Exercises and Mindfulness Activities

10 20 30 40 50 60 70 80 90   ☐ Aerobic   ☐ _____

Time	Intensity/Weights	Activity

Personal activities – Hobbies

_____
_____

Notes: _____
_____

Date:_____

Wake Up	Bed Time	Sleep (HRS)

Diet and Nutrition – Your Food Intake

Breakfast	Lunch
Cal/Pts:	Cal/Pts:
Dinner	**Snack**
Cal/Pts:	Cal/Pts:

Water Intake

How I'm Feeling Today

Physical Exercises and Mindfulness Activities

10 20 30 40 50 60 70 80 90   ☐ Aerobic   ☐ _____

Time	Intensity/Weights	Activity

Personal activities – Hobbies

_____

_____

Notes: _____

Date:_____

Wake Up	Bed Time	Sleep (HRS)

Diet and Nutrition – Your Food Intake

Breakfast	Lunch
Cal/Pts:	Cal/Pts:
Dinner	**Snack**
Cal/Pts:	Cal/Pts:

Water Intake

How I'm Feeling Today

Physical Exercises and Mindfulness Activities

10 20 30 40 50 60 70 80 90   ☐ Aerobic   ☐ _____

Time	Intensity/Weights	Activity

Personal activities – Hobbies

_____
_____

Notes: _____

Date:_____

Wake Up	Bed Time	Sleep (HRS)

Diet and Nutrition – Your Food Intake

Breakfast	Lunch
Cal/Pts:	Cal/Pts:
Dinner	**Snack**
Cal/Pts:	Cal/Pts:

Water Intake

How I'm Feeling Today

Physical Exercises and Mindfulness Activities

10 20 30 40 50 60 70 80 90   ☐ Aerobic ☐ _____

Time	Intensity/Weights	Activity

Personal activities – Hobbies

_____

_____

Notes: _____

KEEP MOVING FORWARD!

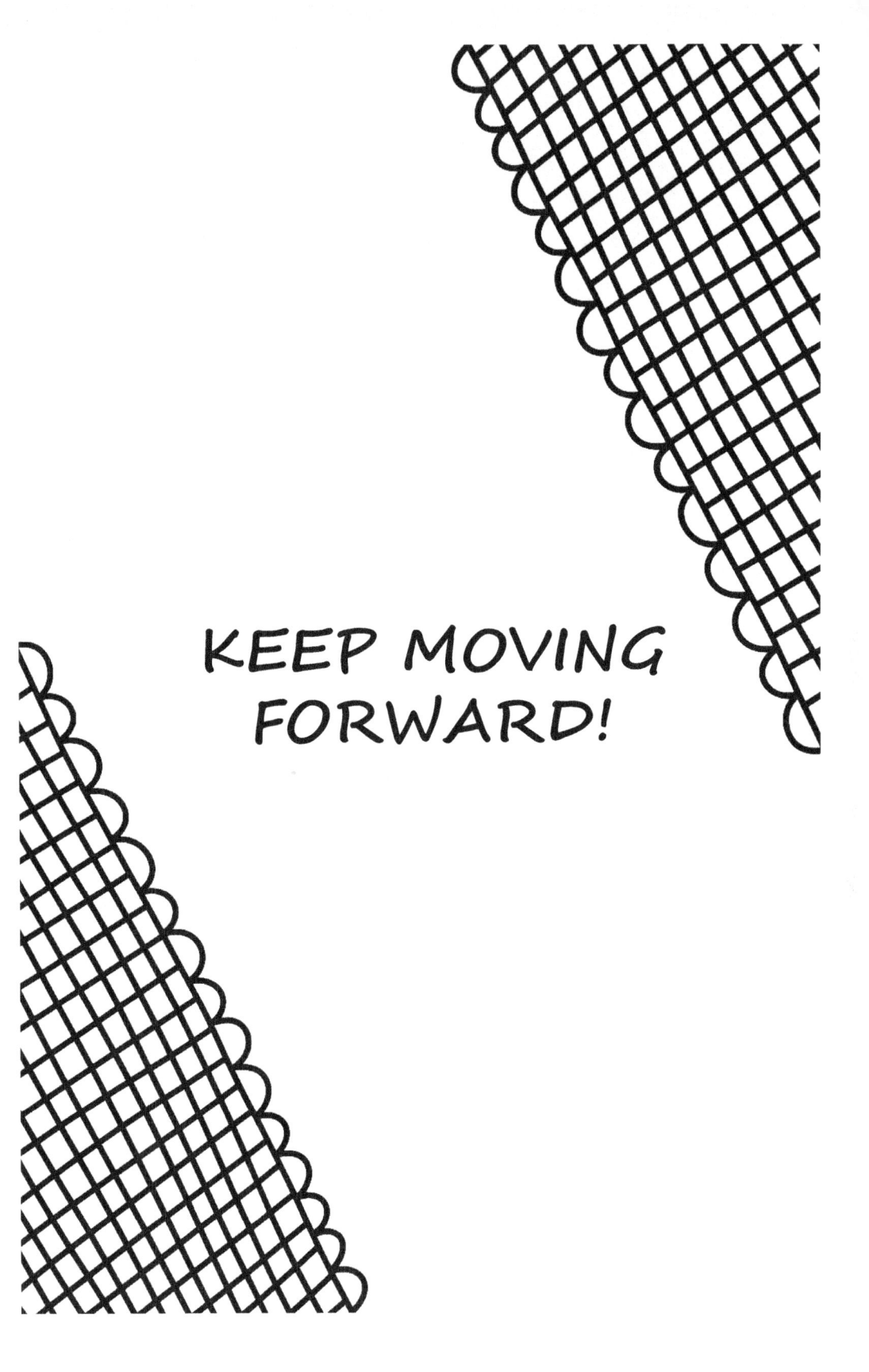

Date:_____

Wake Up	Bed Time	Sleep (HRS)

Diet and Nutrition – Your Food Intake

Breakfast	Lunch
Cal/Pts:	Cal/Pts:
Dinner	**Snack**
Cal/Pts:	Cal/Pts:

Water Intake   How I'm Feeling Today

Physical Exercises and Mindfulness Activities

10 20 30 40 50 60 70 80 90   ☐ Aerobic   ☐ _____

Time	Intensity/Weights	Activity

Personal activities – Hobbies

_____
_____

Notes: _____

Date:_____

Wake Up	Bed Time	Sleep (HRS)

Diet and Nutrition – Your Food Intake

Breakfast	Lunch
Cal/Pts:	Cal/Pts:
Dinner	**Snack**
Cal/Pts:	Cal/Pts:

Water Intake

How I'm Feeling Today

Physical Exercises and Mindfulness Activities

10 20 30 40 50 60 70 80 90   ☐ Aerobic ☐ _____

Time	Intensity/Weights	Activity

Personal activities – Hobbies

_____
_____

Notes: _____

Date:_____

Wake Up	Bed Time	Sleep (HRS)

Diet and Nutrition – Your Food Intake

Breakfast	Lunch
Cal/Pts:	Cal/Pts:
Dinner	**Snack**
Cal/Pts:	Cal/Pts:

Water Intake

How I'm Feeling Today

Physical Exercises and Mindfulness Activities

10 20 30 40 50 60 70 80 90   ☐ Aerobic   ☐ _____

Time	Intensity/Weights	Activity

Personal activities – Hobbies

_____

_____

Notes: _____

Date:_____

Wake Up	Bed Time	Sleep (HRS)

Diet and Nutrition – Your Food Intake

Breakfast	Lunch
Cal/Pts:	Cal/Pts:
Dinner	**Snack**
Cal/Pts:	Cal/Pts:

Water Intake

How I'm Feeling Today

Physical Exercises and Mindfulness Activities

10 20 30 40 50 60 70 80 90 ☐ Aerobic ☐ _____

Time	Intensity/Weights	Activity

Personal activities – Hobbies

_____

_____

Notes: _____

Date:_____

Wake Up	Bed Time	Sleep (HRS)

Diet and Nutrition – Your Food Intake

Breakfast	Lunch
Cal/Pts:	Cal/Pts:
Dinner	**Snack**
Cal/Pts:	Cal/Pts:

Water Intake

How I'm Feeling Today

Physical Exercises and Mindfulness Activities

10 20 30 40 50 60 70 80 90   ☐ Aerobic   ☐ _____

Time	Intensity/Weights	Activity

Personal activities – Hobbies

_____

_____

Notes: _____

Date:_____

Wake Up	Bed Time	Sleep (HRS)

Diet and Nutrition – Your Food Intake

Breakfast	Lunch
Cal/Pts:	Cal/Pts:
Dinner	**Snack**
Cal/Pts:	Cal/Pts:

Water Intake

How I'm Feeling Today

Physical Exercises and Mindfulness Activities

10 20 30 40 50 60 70 80 90 ☐ Aerobic ☐ _____

Time	Intensity/Weights	Activity

Personal activities – Hobbies

_____
_____

Notes: _____
_____

Date:_____

Wake Up	Bed Time	Sleep (HRS)

Diet and Nutrition – Your Food Intake

Breakfast	Lunch
Cal/Pts:	Cal/Pts:
Dinner	**Snack**
Cal/Pts:	Cal/Pts:

Water Intake

How I'm Feeling Today

Physical Exercises and Mindfulness Activities

10 20 30 40 50 60 70 80 90   ☐ Aerobic   ☐ _____

Time	Intensity/Weights	Activity

Personal activities – Hobbies

_____
_____

Notes: _____
_____

GO THAT EXTRA MILE!

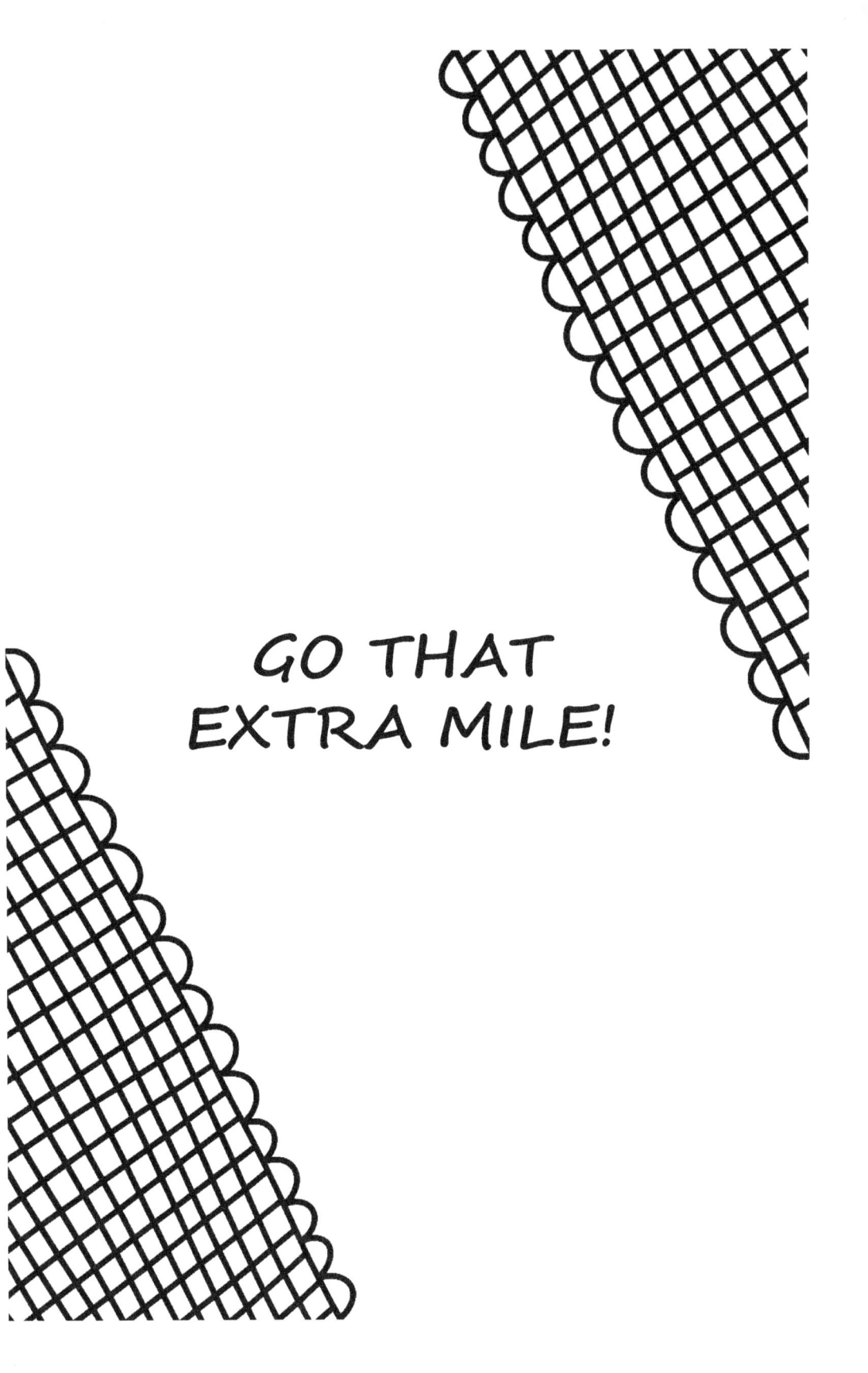

Date:_____

Wake Up	Bed Time	Sleep (HRS)

Diet and Nutrition – Your Food Intake

Breakfast	Lunch
Cal/Pts:	Cal/Pts:
Dinner	**Snack**
Cal/Pts:	Cal/Pts:

Water Intake

How I'm Feeling Today

Physical Exercises and Mindfulness Activities

10 20 30 40 50 60 70 80 90   ☐ Aerobic ☐ _____

Time	Intensity/Weights	Activity

Personal activities – Hobbies

_____

_____

Notes: _____

Date:_____

Wake Up	Bed Time	Sleep (HRS)

Diet and Nutrition – Your Food Intake

Breakfast	Lunch
Cal/Pts:	Cal/Pts:
Dinner	**Snack**
Cal/Pts:	Cal/Pts:

Water Intake

How I'm Feeling Today

Physical Exercises and Mindfulness Activities

10 20 30 40 50 60 70 80 90 ☐ Aerobic ☐ _____

Time	Intensity/Weights	Activity

Personal activities – Hobbies

_____
_____

Notes: _____

Date:_____

Wake Up	Bed Time	Sleep (HRS)

Diet and Nutrition – Your Food Intake

Breakfast	Lunch
Cal/Pts:	Cal/Pts:
Dinner	**Snack**
Cal/Pts:	Cal/Pts:

Water Intake

How I'm Feeling Today

Physical Exercises and Mindfulness Activities

10 20 30 40 50 60 70 80 90   ☐ Aerobic   ☐ _____

Time	Intensity/Weights	Activity

Personal activities – Hobbies

_____

_____

Notes: _____

Date:_____

Wake Up	Bed Time	Sleep (HRS)

Diet and Nutrition – Your Food Intake

Breakfast	Lunch
Cal/Pts:	Cal/Pts:
Dinner	**Snack**
Cal/Pts:	Cal/Pts:

Water Intake   How I'm Feeling Today

Physical Exercises and Mindfulness Activities

10 20 30 40 50 60 70 80 90   ☐ Aerobic   ☐ _____

Time	Intensity/Weights	Activity

Personal activities – Hobbies

_____
_____

Notes: _____

Date:_____

Wake Up	Bed Time	Sleep (HRS)

Diet and Nutrition – Your Food Intake

Breakfast	Lunch
Cal/Pts:	Cal/Pts:
Dinner	**Snack**
Cal/Pts:	Cal/Pts:

Water Intake

How I'm Feeling Today

Physical Exercises and Mindfulness Activities

10 20 30 40 50 60 70 80 90   ☐ Aerobic   ☐ _____

Time	Intensity/Weights	Activity

Personal activities – Hobbies

_____

_____

Notes: _____

Date:_____

Wake Up	Bed Time	Sleep (HRS)

Diet and Nutrition – Your Food Intake

Breakfast	Lunch
Cal/Pts:	Cal/Pts:
Dinner	**Snack**
Cal/Pts:	Cal/Pts:

Water Intake

How I'm Feeling Today

Physical Exercises and Mindfulness Activities

10 20 30 40 50 60 70 80 90   ☐ Aerobic   ☐ _____

Time	Intensity/Weights	Activity

Personal activities – Hobbies

_____
_____

Notes: _____

Date:_____

Wake Up	Bed Time	Sleep (HRS)

Diet and Nutrition – Your Food Intake

Breakfast	Lunch
Cal/Pts:	Cal/Pts:
Dinner	**Snack**
Cal/Pts:	Cal/Pts:

Water Intake

How I'm Feeling Today

Physical Exercises and Mindfulness Activities

10 20 30 40 50 60 70 80 90   ☐ Aerobic   ☐ _____

Time	Intensity/Weights	Activity

Personal activities – Hobbies

_____

_____

Notes: _____

ENJOY LIFE EVERY MOMENT!

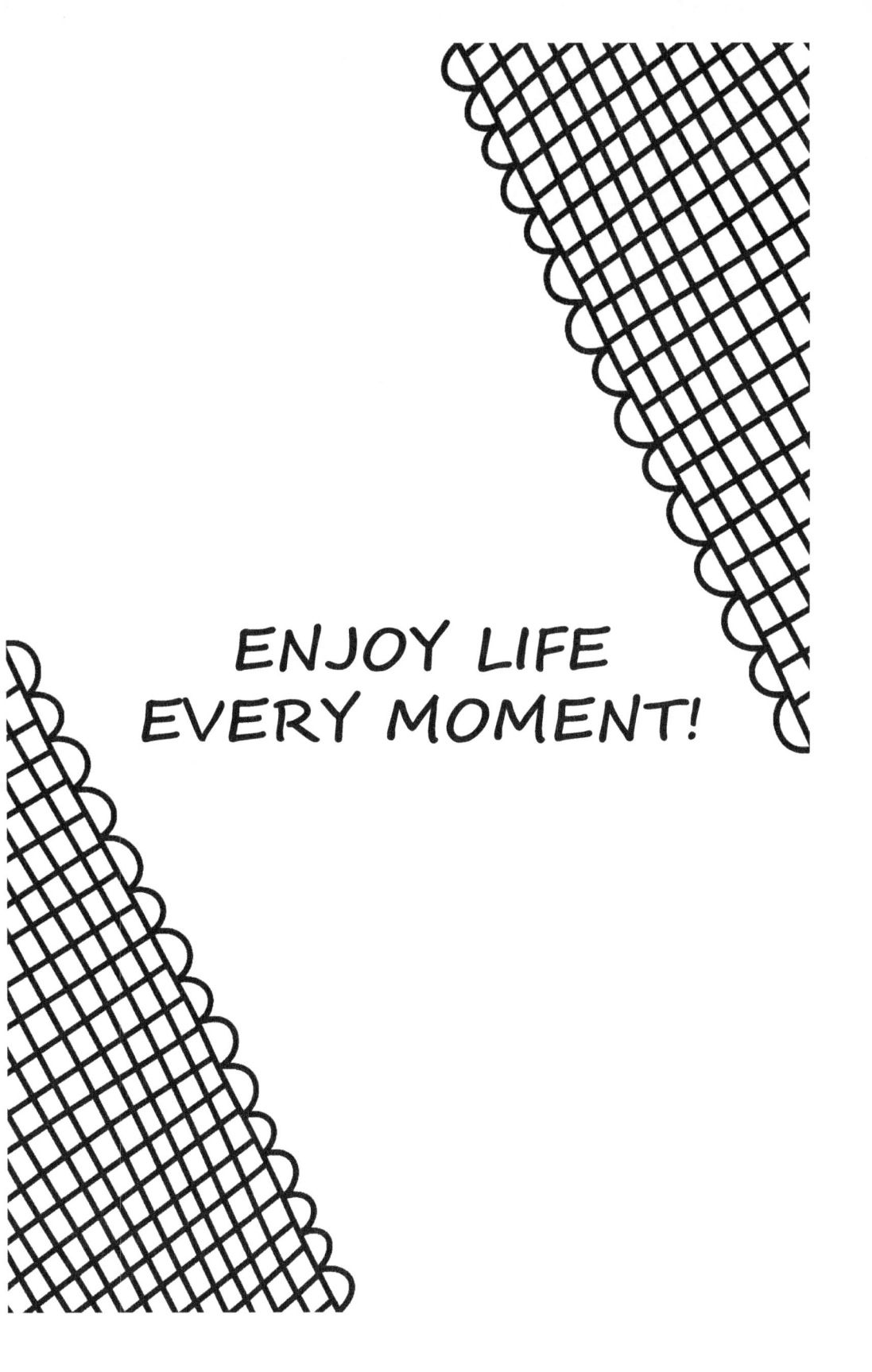

Date:_____

Wake Up	Bed Time	Sleep (HRS)

Diet and Nutrition – Your Food Intake

Breakfast	Lunch
Cal/Pts:	Cal/Pts:

Dinner	Snack
Cal/Pts:	Cal/Pts:

Water Intake

How I'm Feeling Today

Physical Exercises and Mindfulness Activities

10 20 30 40 50 60 70 80 90   ☐ Aerobic ☐ _____

Time	Intensity/Weights	Activity

Personal activities – Hobbies

_____

_____

Notes: _____

Date:_____

Wake Up	Bed Time	Sleep (HRS)

Diet and Nutrition – Your Food Intake

Breakfast	Lunch
Cal/Pts:	Cal/Pts:
Dinner	**Snack**
Cal/Pts:	Cal/Pts:

Water Intake

How I'm Feeling Today

Physical Exercises and Mindfulness Activities

10 20 30 40 50 60 70 80 90   ☐ Aerobic   ☐ _____

Time	Intensity/Weights	Activity

Personal activities – Hobbies

_____
_____

Notes: _____
_____

Date:_____

Wake Up	Bed Time	Sleep (HRS)

Diet and Nutrition – Your Food Intake

Breakfast	Lunch
Cal/Pts:	Cal/Pts:
Dinner	**Snack**
Cal/Pts:	Cal/Pts:

Water Intake   How I'm Feeling Today

Physical Exercises and Mindfulness Activities

10 20 30 40 50 60 70 80 90   ☐ Aerobic   ☐ _____

Time	Intensity/Weights	Activity

Personal activities – Hobbies

_____
_____

Notes: _____

Date:_____

Wake Up	Bed Time	Sleep (HRS)

Diet and Nutrition – Your Food Intake

Breakfast	Lunch
Cal/Pts:	Cal/Pts:
Dinner	**Snack**
Cal/Pts:	Cal/Pts:

Water Intake

How I'm Feeling Today

Physical Exercises and Mindfulness Activities

10 20 30 40 50 60 70 80 90 ☐ Aerobic ☐ _____

Time	Intensity/Weights	Activity

Personal activities – Hobbies

_____
_____

Notes: _____

Date:_____

Wake Up	Bed Time	Sleep (HRS)

Diet and Nutrition – Your Food Intake

Breakfast	Lunch
Cal/Pts:	Cal/Pts:
Dinner	**Snack**
Cal/Pts:	Cal/Pts:

Water Intake

How I'm Feeling Today

Physical Exercises and Mindfulness Activities

10 20 30 40 50 60 70 80 90   ☐ Aerobic   ☐ _____

Time	Intensity/Weights	Activity

Personal activities – Hobbies

_____

_____

Notes: _____

Date:_____

Wake Up	Bed Time	Sleep (HRS)

Diet and Nutrition – Your Food Intake

Breakfast	Lunch
Cal/Pts:	Cal/Pts:
Dinner	**Snack**
Cal/Pts:	Cal/Pts:

Water Intake   How I'm Feeling Today

Physical Exercises and Mindfulness Activities

10 20 30 40 50 60 70 80 90   ☐ Aerobic   ☐ _____

Time	Intensity/Weights	Activity

Personal activities – Hobbies

_____

_____

Notes: _____

Date:_____

Wake Up	Bed Time	Sleep (HRS)

Diet and Nutrition – Your Food Intake

Breakfast	Lunch
Cal/Pts:	Cal/Pts:
Dinner	**Snack**
Cal/Pts:	Cal/Pts:

Water Intake   How I'm Feeling Today

Physical Exercises and Mindfulness Activities

10 20 30 40 50 60 70 80 90   ☐ Aerobic   ☐ _____

Time	Intensity/Weights	Activity

Personal activities – Hobbies

_____

_____

Notes: _____

LITTLE THINGS
MAKE BIG DAYS!

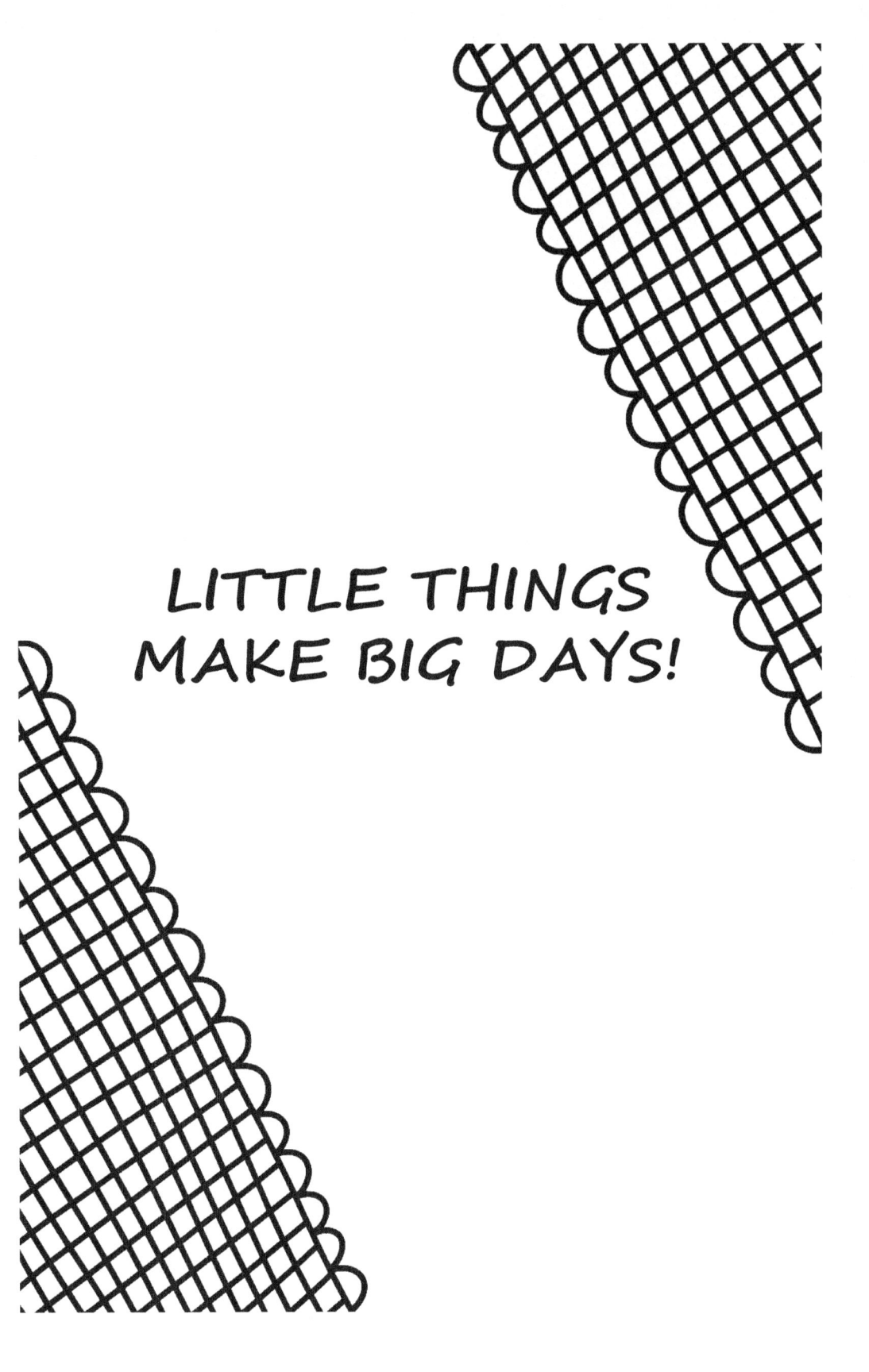

Date:_____

Wake Up	Bed Time	Sleep (HRS)

Diet and Nutrition – Your Food Intake

Breakfast	Lunch
Cal/Pts:	Cal/Pts:
Dinner	**Snack**
Cal/Pts:	Cal/Pts:

Water Intake

How I'm Feeling Today

Physical Exercises and Mindfulness Activities

10 20 30 40 50 60 70 80 90   ☐ Aerobic   ☐ _____

Time	Intensity/Weights	Activity

Personal activities – Hobbies

_____
_____

Notes: _____

Date:_____

Wake Up	Bed Time	Sleep (HRS)

Diet and Nutrition – Your Food Intake

Breakfast	Lunch
Cal/Pts:	Cal/Pts:
Dinner	**Snack**
Cal/Pts:	Cal/Pts:

Water Intake

How I'm Feeling Today

Physical Exercises and Mindfulness Activities

10 20 30 40 50 60 70 80 90   ☐ Aerobic ☐ _____

Time	Intensity/Weights	Activity

Personal activities – Hobbies

_____
_____

Notes: _____

Date:_____

Wake Up	Bed Time	Sleep (HRS)

Diet and Nutrition – Your Food Intake

Breakfast	Lunch
Cal/Pts:	Cal/Pts:
Dinner	**Snack**
Cal/Pts:	Cal/Pts:

Water Intake

How I'm Feeling Today

Physical Exercises and Mindfulness Activities

10 20 30 40 50 60 70 80 90   ☐ Aerobic   ☐ _____

Time	Intensity/Weights	Activity

Personal activities – Hobbies

_____
_____

Notes: _____
_____

Date:_____

Wake Up	Bed Time	Sleep (HRS)

Diet and Nutrition – Your Food Intake

Breakfast	Lunch
Cal/Pts:	Cal/Pts:
Dinner	**Snack**
Cal/Pts:	Cal/Pts:

Water Intake

How I'm Feeling Today

Physical Exercises and Mindfulness Activities

10 20 30 40 50 60 70 80 90   ☐ Aerobic   ☐ _____

Time	Intensity/Weights	Activity

Personal activities – Hobbies

_____
_____

Notes: _____

Date:_____

Wake Up	Bed Time	Sleep (HRS)

Diet and Nutrition – Your Food Intake

Breakfast	Lunch
Cal/Pts:	Cal/Pts:
Dinner	**Snack**
Cal/Pts:	Cal/Pts:

Water Intake

How I'm Feeling Today

Physical Exercises and Mindfulness Activities

10 20 30 40 50 60 70 80 90 ☐ Aerobic ☐ _____

Time	Intensity/Weights	Activity

Personal activities – Hobbies

_____

_____

Notes: _____

Date:_____

Wake Up	Bed Time	Sleep (HRS)

Diet and Nutrition – Your Food Intake

Breakfast	Lunch
Cal/Pts:	Cal/Pts:
Dinner	**Snack**
Cal/Pts:	Cal/Pts:

Water Intake

How I'm Feeling Today

Physical Exercises and Mindfulness Activities

10 20 30 40 50 60 70 80 90 ☐ Aerobic ☐ _____

Time	Intensity/Weights	Activity

Personal activities – Hobbies

_____
_____

Notes: _____

Date:_____

Wake Up	Bed Time	Sleep (HRS)

Diet and Nutrition – Your Food Intake

Breakfast	Lunch
Cal/Pts:	Cal/Pts:
Dinner	**Snack**
Cal/Pts:	Cal/Pts:

Water Intake | How I'm Feeling Today

Physical Exercises and Mindfulness Activities

10 20 30 40 50 60 70 80 90   ☐ Aerobic   ☐ _____

Time	Intensity/Weights	Activity

Personal activities – Hobbies

_____
_____

Notes: _____

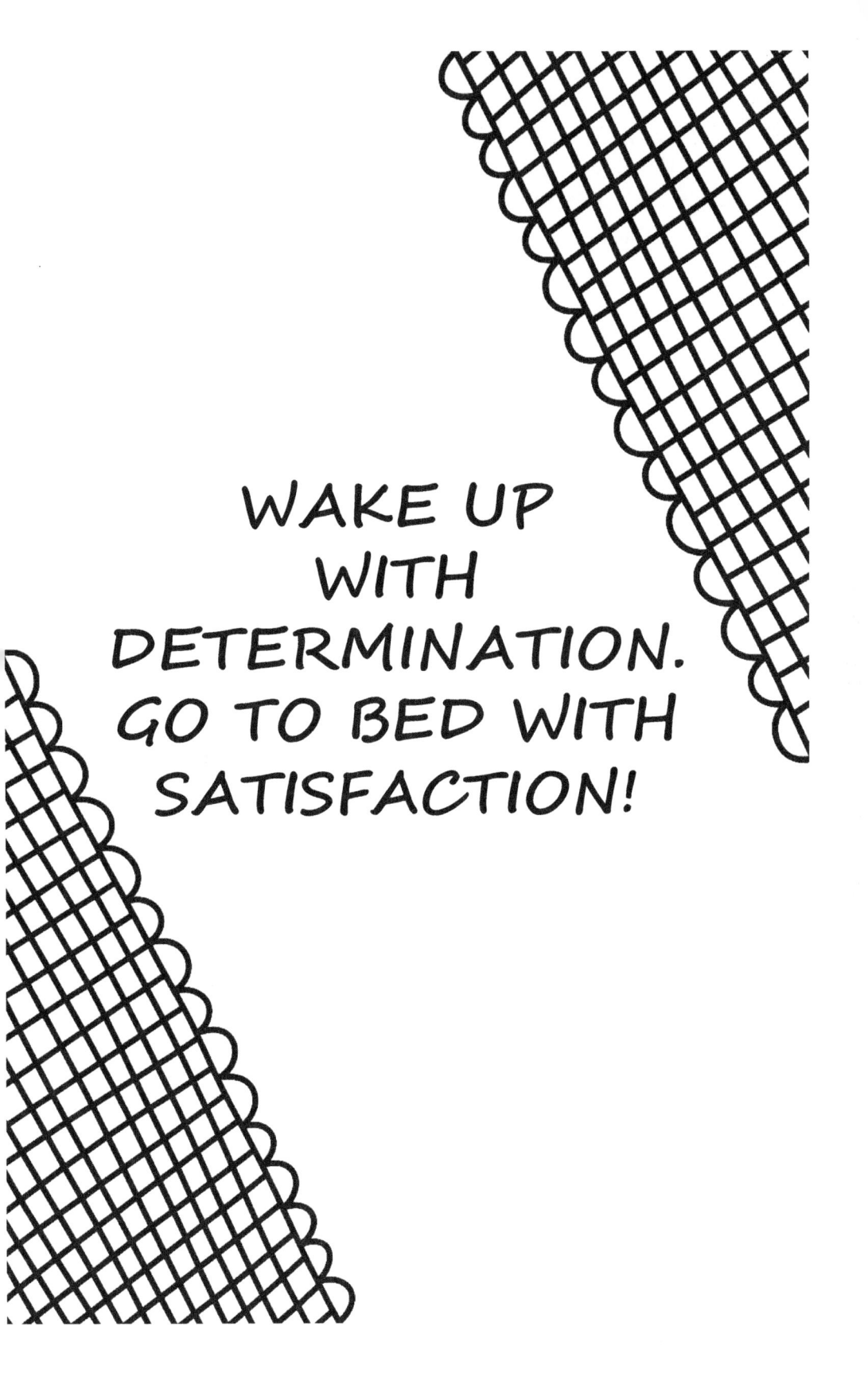

WAKE UP
WITH
DETERMINATION.
GO TO BED WITH
SATISFACTION!

Date:_____

Wake Up	Bed Time	Sleep (HRS)

Diet and Nutrition – Your Food Intake

Breakfast	Lunch
Cal/Pts:	Cal/Pts:
Dinner	**Snack**
Cal/Pts:	Cal/Pts:

Water Intake

How I'm Feeling Today

Physical Exercises and Mindfulness Activities

10 20 30 40 50 60 70 80 90   ☐ Aerobic   ☐ _____

Time	Intensity/Weights	Activity

Personal activities – Hobbies

_____

_____

Notes: _____

Date:_____

Wake Up	Bed Time	Sleep (HRS)

Diet and Nutrition – Your Food Intake

Breakfast	Lunch
Cal/Pts:	Cal/Pts:
Dinner	**Snack**
Cal/Pts:	Cal/Pts:

Water Intake

How I'm Feeling Today

Physical Exercises and Mindfulness Activities

10 20 30 40 50 60 70 80 90   ☐ Aerobic ☐ _____

Time	Intensity/Weights	Activity

Personal activities – Hobbies

_____

_____

Notes: _____

Date:_____

Wake Up	Bed Time	Sleep (HRS)

Diet and Nutrition – Your Food Intake

Breakfast	Lunch
Cal/Pts:	Cal/Pts:
Dinner	**Snack**
Cal/Pts:	Cal/Pts:

Water Intake

How I'm Feeling Today

Physical Exercises and Mindfulness Activities

10 20 30 40 50 60 70 80 90   ☐ Aerobic   ☐ _____

Time	Intensity/Weights	Activity

Personal activities – Hobbies

_____
_____

Notes: _____
_____

Date:_____

Wake Up	Bed Time	Sleep (HRS)

Diet and Nutrition – Your Food Intake

Breakfast	Lunch
Cal/Pts:	Cal/Pts:
Dinner	**Snack**
Cal/Pts:	Cal/Pts:

Water Intake

How I'm Feeling Today

Physical Exercises and Mindfulness Activities

10 20 30 40 50 60 70 80 90   ☐ Aerobic   ☐ _____

Time	Intensity/Weights	Activity

Personal activities – Hobbies

_____
_____

Notes: _____
_____

Date:_____

Wake Up	Bed Time	Sleep (HRS)

Diet and Nutrition – Your Food Intake

Breakfast	Lunch
Cal/Pts:	Cal/Pts:
Dinner	**Snack**
Cal/Pts:	Cal/Pts:

Water Intake

How I'm Feeling Today

Physical Exercises and Mindfulness Activities

10 20 30 40 50 60 70 80 90   ☐ Aerobic   ☐ _____

Time	Intensity/Weights	Activity

Personal activities – Hobbies

_____

_____

Notes: _____

Date:_____

Wake Up	Bed Time	Sleep (HRS)

Diet and Nutrition – Your Food Intake

Breakfast	Lunch
Cal/Pts:	Cal/Pts:
Dinner	**Snack**
Cal/Pts:	Cal/Pts:

Water Intake
How I'm Feeling Today

Physical Exercises and Mindfulness Activities

10 20 30 40 50 60 70 80 90   ☐ Aerobic   ☐ _____

Time	Intensity/Weights	Activity

Personal activities – Hobbies

_____
_____

Notes: _____

Date:_____

Wake Up	Bed Time	Sleep (HRS)

Diet and Nutrition – Your Food Intake

Breakfast	Lunch
Cal/Pts:	Cal/Pts:
Dinner	**Snack**
Cal/Pts:	Cal/Pts:

Water Intake

How I'm Feeling Today

Physical Exercises and Mindfulness Activities

10 20 30 40 50 60 70 80 90   ☐ Aerobic   ☐ _____

Time	Intensity/Weights	Activity

Personal activities – Hobbies

_____

_____

Notes: _____

WORK HARD,
DREAM BIG,
NEVER GIVE UP!

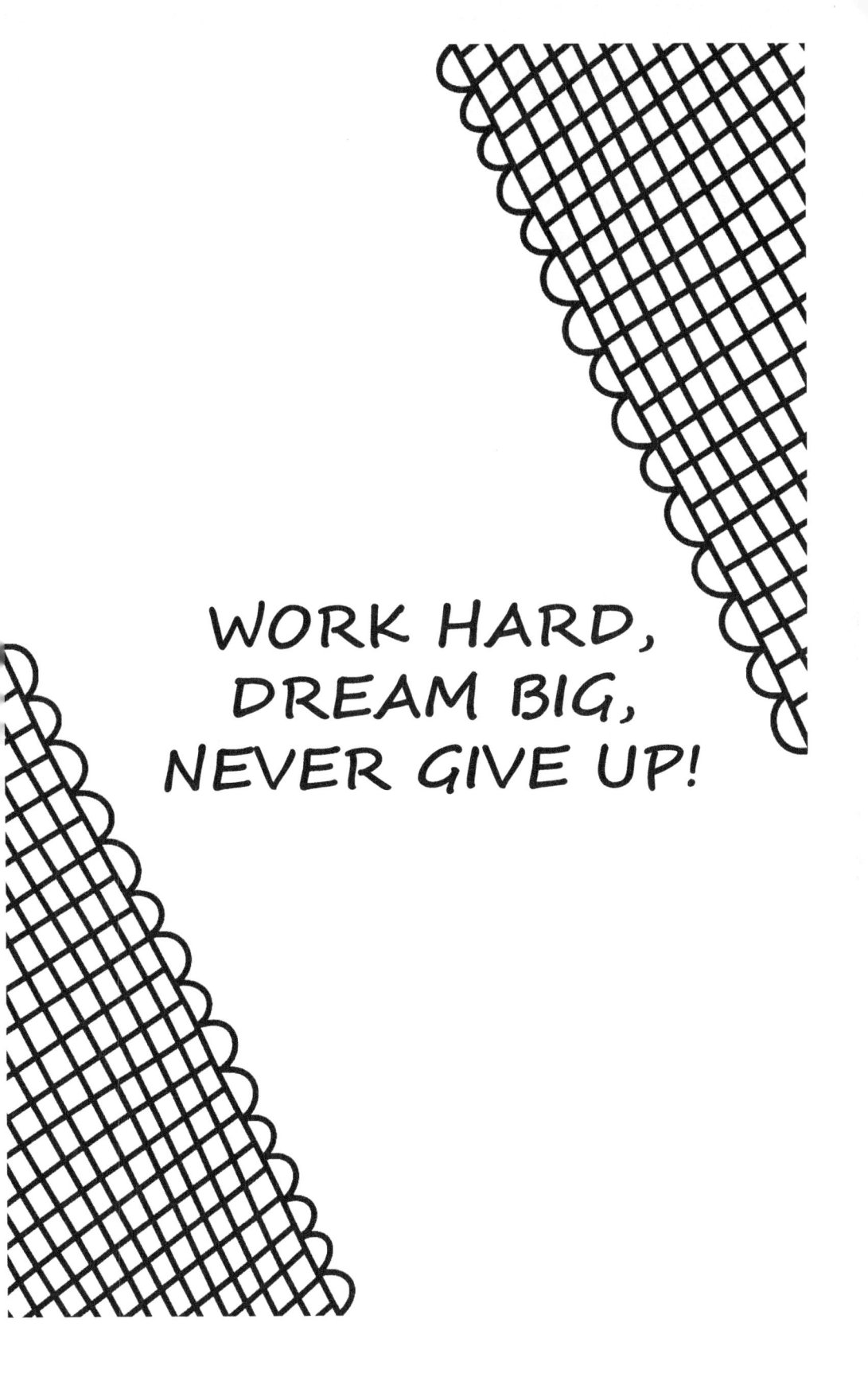

Date:_____

Wake Up	Bed Time	Sleep (HRS)

Diet and Nutrition – Your Food Intake

Breakfast	Lunch
Cal/Pts:	Cal/Pts:
Dinner	**Snack**
Cal/Pts:	Cal/Pts:

Water Intake

How I'm Feeling Today

Physical Exercises and Mindfulness Activities

10 20 30 40 50 60 70 80 90   ☐ Aerobic   ☐ _____

Time	Intensity/Weights	Activity

Personal activities – Hobbies

_____

_____

Notes: _____

Date:_____

Wake Up	Bed Time	Sleep (HRS)

Diet and Nutrition – Your Food Intake

Breakfast	Lunch
Cal/Pts:	Cal/Pts:
Dinner	Snack
Cal/Pts:	Cal/Pts:

Water Intake

How I'm Feeling Today

Physical Exercises and Mindfulness Activities

10 20 30 40 50 60 70 80 90   ☐ Aerobic   ☐ _____

Time	Intensity/Weights	Activity

Personal activities – Hobbies

_____

_____

Notes: _____

Date:_____

Wake Up	Bed Time	Sleep (HRS)

Diet and Nutrition – Your Food Intake

Breakfast	Lunch
Cal/Pts:	Cal/Pts:
Dinner	**Snack**
Cal/Pts:	Cal/Pts:

Water Intake   How I'm Feeling Today

Physical Exercises and Mindfulness Activities

10 20 30 40 50 60 70 80 90   ☐ Aerobic   ☐ _____

Time	Intensity/Weights	Activity

Personal activities – Hobbies

_____
_____

Notes: _____

Date:_____

Wake Up	Bed Time	Sleep (HRS)

Diet and Nutrition – Your Food Intake

Breakfast	Lunch
Cal/Pts:	Cal/Pts:
Dinner	**Snack**
Cal/Pts:	Cal/Pts:

Water Intake   How I'm Feeling Today

Physical Exercises and Mindfulness Activities

10 20 30 40 50 60 70 80 90   ☐ Aerobic ☐ _____

Time	Intensity/Weights	Activity

Personal activities – Hobbies

_____
_____

Notes: _____
_____

Date:_____

Wake Up	Bed Time	Sleep (HRS)

Diet and Nutrition – Your Food Intake

Breakfast	Lunch
Cal/Pts:	Cal/Pts:
Dinner	**Snack**
Cal/Pts:	Cal/Pts:

Water Intake

How I'm Feeling Today

Physical Exercises and Mindfulness Activities

10 20 30 40 50 60 70 80 90   ☐ Aerobic ☐ _____

Time	Intensity/Weights	Activity

Personal activities – Hobbies

_____
_____

Notes: _____

Date:_____

Wake Up	Bed Time	Sleep (HRS)

Diet and Nutrition – Your Food Intake

Breakfast	Lunch
Cal/Pts:	Cal/Pts:
Dinner	**Snack**
Cal/Pts:	Cal/Pts:

Water Intake

How I'm Feeling Today

Physical Exercises and Mindfulness Activities

10 20 30 40 50 60 70 80 90   ☐ Aerobic   ☐ _____

Time	Intensity/Weights	Activity

Personal activities – Hobbies

_____
_____

Notes: _____
_____

Date:_____

Wake Up	Bed Time	Sleep (HRS)

Diet and Nutrition – Your Food Intake

Breakfast	Lunch
Cal/Pts:	Cal/Pts:
Dinner	**Snack**
Cal/Pts:	Cal/Pts:

Water Intake 　　　　How I'm Feeling Today

Physical Exercises and Mindfulness Activities

10 20 30 40 50 60 70 80 90   ☐ Aerobic   ☐ _____

Time	Intensity/Weights	Activity

Personal activities – Hobbies

_____

_____

Notes: _____

BE PROUD OF YOURSELF!

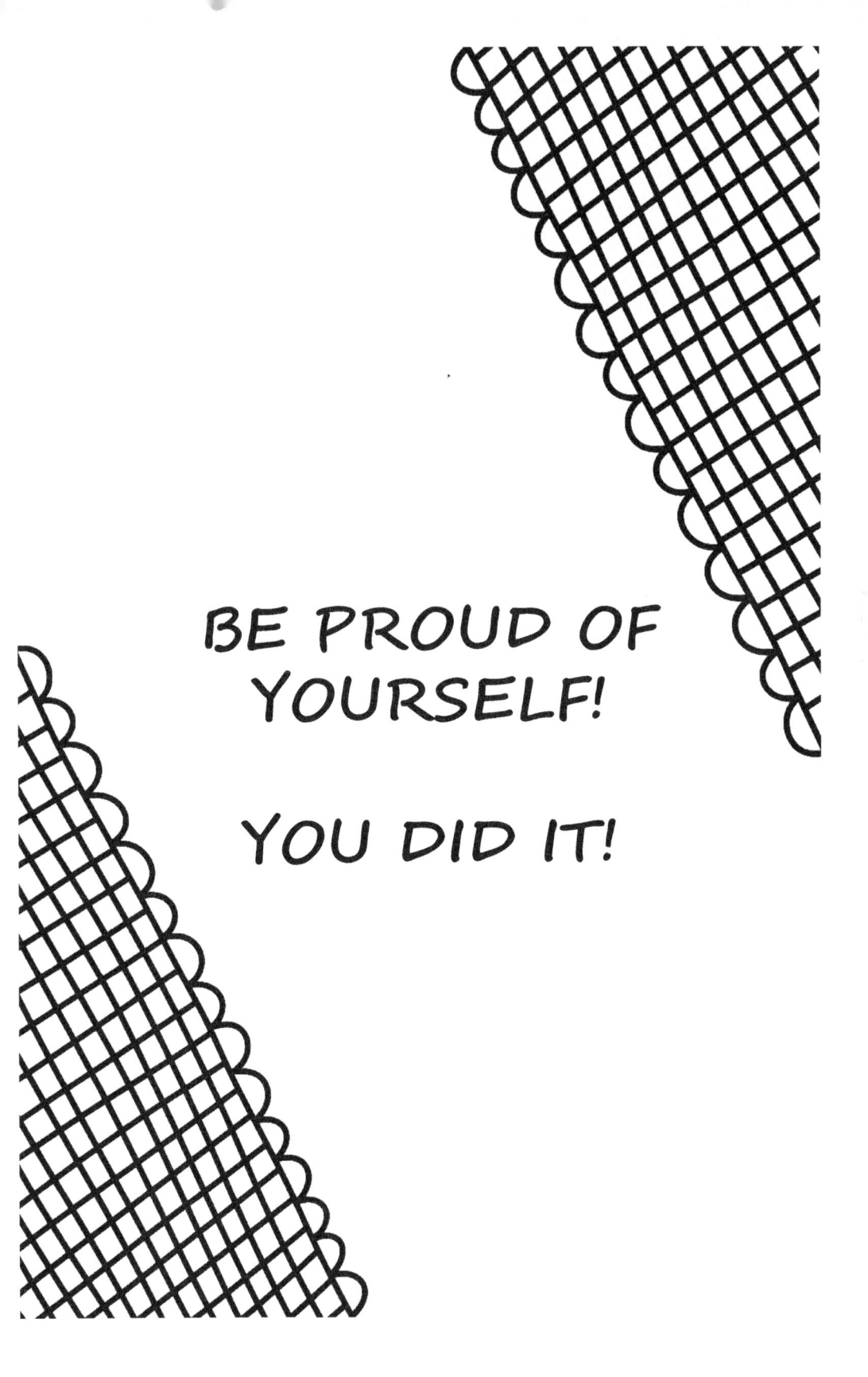

YOU DID IT!

Date:_____

Wake Up	Bed Time	Sleep (HRS)

Diet and Nutrition – Your Food Intake

Breakfast	Lunch
Cal/Pts:	Cal/Pts:
Dinner	**Snack**
Cal/Pts:	Cal/Pts:

Water Intake

How I'm Feeling Today

Physical Exercises and Mindfulness Activities

10 20 30 40 50 60 70 80 90 ☐ Aerobic ☐ _____

Time	Intensity/Weights	Activity

Personal activities – Hobbies

_____
_____

Notes: _____

Date:_____

Wake Up	Bed Time	Sleep (HRS)

Diet and Nutrition – Your Food Intake

Breakfast	Lunch
Cal/Pts:	Cal/Pts:
Dinner	**Snack**
Cal/Pts:	Cal/Pts:

Water Intake

How I'm Feeling Today

Physical Exercises and Mindfulness Activities

10 20 30 40 50 60 70 80 90   ☐ Aerobic   ☐ _____

Time	Intensity/Weights	Activity

Personal activities – Hobbies

_____

_____

Notes: _____

Printed in Great Britain
by Amazon